Glitter

Real Stories
From Real Women
About Sexual Desire

Edited by Mona Darling

TO MY MAL

To my best friend and favorite bartender. Fourteen plus years of stalking and you still haven't been able to ditch me! Thank you for putting up with my incredibly weird career choice.

Had I the dare to choose, I'd choose you from all the men on all the planets the night sky has to show me.

Saffron (Christina Hendricks), *Firefly*

INTRODUCING THE GLITTER GIRLS

ACKNOWLEDGMENTS

I want to thank every woman who shared her story. By opening up and sharing your fantasies and desires, you are normalizing and de-stigmatizing women's sex and desire.

You are all amazing.

I also want to thank everyone who encouraged me to continue collecting these stories. It has been a true labor of love.

A portion of all proceeds is donated to a certain large women's health organization that neither knows about, nor endorses this book.

Glitter

Foreword

When I started my blog, talking about IVF, parenting, and my job as a dominatrix, I wasn't sure what to expect. I thought I might get hate mail from people who didn't understand that sex workers and BDSM players could be loving parents. I expected to be shunned by the other mommy bloggers. But instead, they welcomed me. I shared their same struggles with parenting and infertility, yet was able to talk to them about another side of themselves that they usually kept private. Women from every walk of life started telling me about their secret desires and past adventures, their sexual histories.

At first I talked to these women privately. Some talked about kinky escapades 'back in the day,' while others confessed things they had never shared before: a rape or particularly shaming curiosity that had affected their sex lives. Most didn't want an answer, they just wanted to be heard; to talk to someone who wouldn't judge. To feel like they weren't alone.

We all think we are alone. We are the only one. That we need to hide that part of us. In reality? We all have a past: a desire, a fetish, a kink, a secret.

This book is a collection of those secret stories.

Some are sexual histories taking the reader down a path of relevant events that brought the writer to where she is today. Some are stories about one particular event or relationship, be it tragic, kinky or hot. The one thing that brings them all together is that they are all true stories from real women.

Reading these stories feels like exchanging secrets with a room full of girlfriends over cocktails. Many cocktails.

I want this anthology to be a talking point, a conversation starter. I want any woman who reads it to come away from the book identifying with at least one story; to know that they are not alone, to feel less ashamed and more empowered.

The contributors to this anthology discuss everything from masturbation to fetishes, from sexy to sad. Not every story will sit well with you for a variety of reasons. I hope you can still read it and be supportive of the writers.

LET THE GLITTER BEGIN!

TEXTUALLY ACTIVE

Amber

@AFullMargin

I'm a full time single parent and full time student preparing to transfer into my first bachelors program at thirty. I'm pansexual, kinky and tend to avoid politics and religion wherever I can. I'm a bad feminist. I've been writing fanfiction and erotica for over fifteen years and, at the moment it's my sexual outlet of choice.

I came of age in the '90s, born in 1982 and raised in rural Arizona by working parents that didn't really think I needed sex ed - they were right, by the time they thought to even begin introducing it at school and eventually at home I was already prepared for the advanced courses. Bless a precocious mind and easy access to pornography.

After dinner, I put the kids to bed, light a few candles and some mellow-scented incense. A mug of tea, usually lavender or mint, and something sweet to nibble on complete my personal self-care regimen. Before I had kids, it'd be my boyfriend or girlfriend going to bed and when I used to drink, it'd be a shallow tumbler with a double shot of tequila instead of tea and when I smoked it'd be my trusty Marlboro hard pack and zippo instead of hand-dipped incense, but the routine has remained mostly unchanged for over a decade. I turn on my computer and with a few keystrokes the experience has begun.

Tonight, I'm a bubbly twenty-six-year-old vixen looking to wrap my fingers around a sugar daddy's big fat...wallet by the best means at my easy disposal, this time by posing as an escort. Yesterday I was a wealthy executive being beaten and fucked raw by an ex-commando mercenary working for a man that I screwed on a business deal. Maybe tomorrow I'll go off my rails and change into the hazy green skin of a tentacle monster on the hunt for virgins who dare disturb my slumber. Perhaps I'll be a fifty-something divorcee meeting with his new lady love for a clandestine night of passion between slices of his homemade pie and full contact cuddling. Or even a super-spy bedding an intersexed space alien he met in a pandimensional brothel, an awkward thirty-something with an unspoken crush on his long-time best friend, a bored plus-sized housewife who decides to moonlight as a mistress for thrills, any number of gawky young adults still learning about the pleasures of sex, a survivor of the zombie apocalypse desperate to feel anything but fear and hopelessness, a curious anthropomorphic feline, part of a gang bang, a sex slave or slave owner. I could be anything, any one, any number of faces and bodies and stories working toward the simple goal of text on the screen dripping with unadulterated lust.

This is my sex. Late at night by the light of a few candles and my monitor I spin stories of sex and intrigue, lust and longing. Tales where lonely cops, waitresses, mythical creatures, parents, teenagers, models, politicians, soldiers and spies are stripped down to the level of lovers. Givers and takers, tops and bottoms, masters, mistresses, slaves and pets and anything and everything in between. My fantasies, no matter how taboo or vanilla they are that day, are safe and as free from judgement as one can be while still straying out of the solid walls of my mind.

Far from what I've been told people assume when they find out about my text-based hobbies, I've had sex in the real world. Quite a bit of it, considering I'm a fairly unassuming looking overweight thirty-year-old single mom. I started young, too young, perhaps, but curiosity has always gotten the better of me and over the last fifteen years I've dabbled in anything that's taken my interest. Much like my fantasy life, finding my true self IRL (in real life) has been difficult. The list of identities I've held in one form or another includes (but is certainly not limited to): bisexual, gender queer, victim, bottom, mistress, gay, goddess, top, slave, slut, boi, little girl, ftm, observer, furry, director. Right now, at this moment, I consider myself to be a pansexual mamabear with toppy tendencies despite my intensely submissive fantasies...it's a label that's stuck longer than most but I won't pretend it's how I'll always see myself.

The 'vanilla' world disappointed me, I remember as a young teenager being frustrated with the pervasive reliance on gender roles and rigid "gay" or "straight" sexuality. The black-and-white world of this-is-good/that-is-bad has always bothered me and the only way I could ever explain it is to say that my world is gray. Which in and of itself isn't entirely true. It's more like it's a Technicolor rainbow of possibilities where things are flexible and fluid and the rigid notion of sexuality being an either/or only continuum was done away with. Throughout my formative years I can remember the streams of contradictory information coming from every direction: girls only like boys but good girls don't sleep with boys and you should have a close female friend but if you kiss you're lesbians and that's dirty...

I forged my own way. I played with boys and girls, exploring everything I could, like a fat kid at a Dairy Queen with a big bowl of little pink spoons (which was also a literal indulgence of mine, but in all fairness I was a pretty cool fat kid). Before too long, though, *they* took my spoons away and I was left without people to explore. At thirteen I was the weird kid who giggled a lot and knew way too much about sex: the pervert and the slut. That was the year I started writing.

The first gentle steps into textual sexuality were much like the fumblings of any virgin; I kept a diary where I wrote down all of my fantasies in gory, graphic detail. Thoughts I'm almost ashamed to admit came out of the mind of a sexually-obsessed tween. Things along the lines of "I bet Mr. (insert teacher here) has a really big dick. I wonder what would happen if I told him I'd suck it." Which – oddly enough – would be one of my first documented fantasies involving intergenerational relationships with an authority figure, something which has popped up many, many times in my fantasies since. At fourteen I fell in love with the internet and found fanfiction, which I still write to this day and don't ever plan to stop. I've just this year found my very first stories under a pseudonym I haven't used since 1999. In them Hercules and Ioalus (from TV's *Hercules: the Legendary Journeys*) shared a very manly time at the baths including scrubbing and copious amounts of poorly-written anal sex. Many stories followed, all based in various fandoms and around various pairings.

After those initial writings I became like a woman possessed. I wrote about anything and everything, spending hours chatting with friends who were into the same exact things I was. It was heavenly but at that time it was all limited to discussing *fictional* sex lives. It was safe but unsatisfying. I got my personal kicks in the real world, experimenting with sex all through high school with anyone I was attracted to that seemed interested in me. I supplemented heavily with porn in every form I could get my hands on: videos, magazines, books, nifty.org and newsgroups with alt.sex in them.

My next big step in my personal textual-sexual revolution came in the form of something anyone who has ever been in a large chatroom has probably seen: an instant message with the simple line "a/s/l." I can't remember the guy's handle, but shortly after I answered it became pretty clear what he wanted. Eventually he asked outright what my fantasy was, and for the first time ever I shared my biggest fantasy of the time: for a marching band practice (I would be the third chair trombone in this scenario) to turn into an orgy. Oddly enough, it's one of the few fantasies that has survived to this day and every so often I'll Google 'marching band orgy' only to be sorely disappointed and reminded that when I die some poor soul will end up reading my search history and learning things nobody ever needed to know. In return, he sent a grainy webcam picture of his cock. Thus began the cybersex portion of my sexual journey.

Cybersex was my first introduction to openly sharing my own fantasies, learning about kinks that I had always assumed nobody but me had. I'd stay up until the early hours of the morning getting off with men and women I never intended to meet, sharing our fantasies over IM and in private chatrooms, one-on-one or in small groups. In that time I was always upfront about who I was, no characters, just a lonely, horny girl looking to swap fantasies and talk about the weird shit I'd love to do with someone else. The cybersex led to real life sex back then, random hookups and my shaky introductions to the BDSM scene around eighteen or nineteen when I was treated horribly for being a newbie and more or less clueless about things like roles or identities; I just wanted to play! And I played. And learned games that I hadn't even thought about at that point in my life. I recall on my twentieth birthday I got my very first caning at a play party because I'd mentioned to a guy I met in a chatroom that I wondered what it would feel like to be beaten and humiliated and then fucked in public. I got to play out fantasies of being "Daddy's girl" as well as a mistress with a man twice my age licking my toes before begging to eat me out. It was a pretty good run, really. But in the end, it was just too much. I got sick of being told I *had* to be either a Domme or a sub, that I *had* to be into leather and pain and humiliation, which sometimes I was, but not always. But again, there were always those either/or lines. Too many times I got told that situational switches don't exist or that I wasn't straight enough or that I wasn't lesbian enough or that it was a man- or woman-only space. I got sick of fucking people I barely knew and engaging in what I now know was very risky and self-destructive behavior and plain old poor judgement. I wanted freedom to not just be me, but to be anyone I damn well pleased. And I wanted to be loved for it.

Retreating back to the internet, I found a place to call home, the furthest place I could possibly find from the leather-and-pain I thought of as BDSM at the time: I became a furry. Okay, to clarify: I've never been sexually attracted to animals, nor do I ever expect to be. I never wore a fursuit (though I have played with someone in one) and I never subscribed the whole 'otherkin' thing. That said, for a (before-children) period between the ages of about twenty-one and twenty-three I identified as an anthropomorphic gray and black tabby cat. Still with me? Good, you're a trooper.

The furry community was an eye-opener for me, for the first time I found others that were in tune with my philosophy of sexuality as something that should be playful and friendly (even when the scene you're playing isn't). I was able to explore fluctuating identities and the concept of playing a character other than myself in a sexual context. My writing changed and grew as I did until it too became more fluid. Fiction began to crossover into my life as cybersex with the intent to get off and maybe hook up with someone was replaced with roleplay where the goal was to weave a story with someone else.

But again, I grew and changed and my sexuality and identity changed with me. Over the course of the next five years I'd have two lovely children, become a single parent, and lose most interest in actually having sex with someone in the real world. Don't get me wrong, if the right person and the right time happened to coincide, I wouldn't think twice about it, but most days I'm pretty sure I've had more than my share of the ice cream buffet that is sex.

Roleplay and fiction became my outlet of choice then, and for over three years now I've been pretty happy with that. My sex life is far from over, in a lot of ways I see it as just beginning in this world where I can be anyone I can imagine and indulge in things I either can't or wouldn't do in the real world. If I wanted to, tonight I could be Batman. I could write a story by myself or with friends where I yet again save Gotham and then have a three-way with Catwoman and Robin. Leaving the masks on, of course. And if I feel like it, I can be an unassuming thirty-year-old single mom with a wild imagination who wants to cuddle and maybe kiss and someday fall in love. It's like a pornographic costume party where we're all wearing a mask and our readers (of what we choose to make public) are voyeurs to our exhibitionism.

At the end of the night, when my lust is sated and my imagination has drifted off, I snuff out my candles and shut down my computer before retiring to bed with a few good toys and a very, very vivid memory of the many lives I lead.

THE SNOW STORM

Christy Summer

I'm a thirty-something wife and mom who previously partied like a rock star and has all the memories to prove it. I had a strict religious upbringing and let it all go when I hit my twenties. I can currently be found reading books to my toddlers, relaxing at a local bar or writing about my previous party life.

I knew what I wanted when I drove to the mall that night. I didn't care that it was snowing like hell outside and that the parking lots were iced over. I wanted him and I wasn't sure when I'd see him again.

We both knew that it was risky, but I for one did not care. All I wanted was to experience his hands on me, sense his tongue tracing the inside of my lips and to feel him inside me again. It was all I'd thought about that afternoon at work, after he'd brought lunch to me and I'd sat next to him, having to control myself when all I had wanted was to fuck him, right there, in his truck.

Later I found out that originally his intentions for that night had not included sex, but of course he didn't protest when I got on top of him. I could not help myself. Five minutes of kissing him, feeling his hands touch me, first over my skirt, then pushing my skirt up and out of the way so that he could grab my hip, and then finally slide his fingers inside me, where I was already so wet and so ready that I was moaning - I simply couldn't wait any longer.

I had to have him, right there in the parking lot, in a snow storm, in his truck. I got on top of him and positioned myself so that I could feel every inch of him.

I still remember everything about that night: how amazing he felt inside me, the scent of his sweat mixed with mine, his hands, grabbing my hips to pull himself deeper into me; the feel of his mouth on my neck, my collarbone, finally my own mouth, kissing me with a passionate but controlled need. The excitement of possibly getting caught made everything more intense. The look in his eyes when we came up for air, the sound of his voice and the feeling of his breath on my neck: he's a vocal lover, something that turns me on so incredibly quickly. I never had to wonder if I felt good to him, his words and moans told me everything.

We completely fogged up his truck that night and were both left dripping, covered with the sweet smell of sex. I had come three times and was blissfully exhausted. There were more times between us after that, but something about that particular time was different. Maybe it was the contrast of the cold outside and the hot, sweaty sex inside the truck. Perhaps it was the intensity with which I had to have him. Whatever it was, that night is now one that I will never forget.

If I'm Going To Be Honest...

Courtney

I'm in my thirties and I'm studying for my masters in psychology. I am also a homeschooling single mother.

I'm going to go ahead and say it; I like to watch gay

male porn. I mean *really* like it. Nothing gets me as turned on as seeing a ripped, sweaty man taking it from another hot man.

I wasn't always this way, although I have always been a little...*outside* of the normal bounds of sexuality. I have had a history of experimenting with some lite BDSM, always in role as the submissive. Long ago I discovered, while wrestling with a male friend, that it really turned me on to be pinned down and helpless. I got so wet from that experience, it was embarrassing. I have always played the subservient, docile woman. Even when watching porn, it was always of some submissive, busty blonde being subjugated by a strict, dominant man.

I have been tied up, had sensory deprivation, been spanked and whipped, and been called a 'dirty little slut' more times than I can count.

However, after recently ending a particularly difficult long-term romantic relationship that was borderline emotionally abusive, it suddenly repulsed me to see women being taken advantage of in porn, regardless of whether or not it is fictional. I could not imagine playing the submissive role ever again, even knowing that it is just a role I am playing. My whole sexual viewpoint has been flipped upside down. But, instead of feeling lost and being upset at this upheaval, I am embracing the prospect and using it to explore the multitudes of other options that are out there for me in the sexual rainbow.

I might expand my porn viewing to women fucking men with strap-ons or women fucking women with strap-ons. I love that there are so many options to express sexuality and vow never to limit myself to the submissive box again. The idea that men can be the submissive or even just the bottom excites the hell out of me. I might even give domination a go in my next sexual relationship.

For now, I will enjoy watching hot men fucking, and I will do so without shame!

AFTER SCHOOL SPECIAL

Alicia Wolfe

A wine connoisseur with an amazing rack and a dog of an ex-husband. She leads a pretty normal life as a number cruncher, wife and mom/slave to three cats.

Apparently I was rather young the first time I had sex. That's what people tell me when they hear 'my number' anyway. It didn't feel that young to me at the time. I was fourteen. It was 1988.

What did I know about sex at the time? Plenty. A friend had given me *The Joy of Sex* as a gag gift. And I had studied it. Prior to that, aside from the basic mechanics, the only instruction I had had on sex I'd gotten "on the street" because all my mother had to say was "Sex is a very wonderful and beautiful thing between two married people."

I put that in quotes because I remember it verbatim. Because she said it in those exact words over and over again. It was actually more like, "SexIsAVery-WonderfulAndBeautifulThingBetweenTwoMarried-People."

Spoken in monotone.

That was it.

Unlike other first time stories I've heard, I wasn't pressured by the guy to do it, at least not in the traditional sense of "C'mon, baby, let's do it. You're giving me blue balls." It was my idea.

In retrospect, it was not one of my better ideas.

But I don't regret it. I have always been one to go my own way and this experience was no exception.

My boyfriend at the time, let's call him Mike to protect the stupid, was clearly more...um...'experienced' than me. I suppose I was "the good girl" to his "bad boy," he did have a mohawk after all. But he actually didn't try much with me when we would make out. I do remember him once trying to finger me while we were kissing and I gently moved his hand away ... because I had my period.

Ew, gross!

But I didn't tell him that. How embarrassing.

He never tried anything else 'underneath clothing'. He behaved like a gentleman in that regard. I remember thinking that was odd. I wanted to try more, experience more. Or find out that I didn't by saying 'no' if he tried something I wasn't ready for. But that one act of pushing his hand away had apparently sealed my fate.

Then came a time, perhaps a month or two later, when I didn't see him for a week or two. I think I was grounded. I was pretty much always grounded because my crazy mother *thought* I was out partying, boozing and having sex. It probably had something to do with the fact that she had found that book hidden in my dresser. But I wasn't doing any of that. My mother drove me everywhere I went. She called parents before I went wherever she drove me. She was completely delusional in her accusations.

I can't remember which came first, the rumor about Mike and another girl or a close friend telling me she had lost her cherry. I don't think it really matters which. The point was, I now had a really good friend who had 'done it.' And I had a boyfriend who apparently *wanted* to do 'it' and was perhaps doing 'it' with someone else because he thought I wouldn't do 'it'.

I decided to find out what 'it' was all about. Being a fourteen-year-old girl, of course, I also did 'it' thinking 'it' would help me keep my man. That reason makes me want to kick my former self now. That is the stupidest reason possible and if my mother had only had a real conversation with me about sex...

I told him I wanted to do 'it' and I conspired to be somewhere I wasn't supposed to be (divorced parents can be useful that way: "didn't she stay at *your* house last night?"). And we did it.

It was...painful, I guess. I've heard many describe it as traumatic. Not for me. It just...was. It hurt. He tried to back out of it because it was hard to um...ya know...insert tab A into slot B. Especially with a condom on (I may have been young and naïve but I sure wasn't stupid). There was pretty much zero foreplay. I'm sure there must have been blood but I don't specifically remember that. He was nice enough about it. And he clearly was *not* as experienced as I had thought he was. He might have done it before but it was clear he hadn't had much practice.

There was quite a lot of fumbling around. We were in someone's empty spare room. I think we just had blankets and a sleeping bag, maybe. I don't think there was even a mattress on the floor. Romantic it was not. A tender moment? Nope. It was more like research.

For my part, I just wanted to do it. Get it over with. Find out what was the big deal. And what I found out was...it wasn't that big a deal. I didn't love it. I didn't hate it.

He didn't speak to me after that.

I got away with that rendezvous as far as my mother was concerned but then I think I was punished for some other made up transgression. And so I finally came to the (inevitable) conclusion that if I was gonna do the time, I might as well do the crime. Especially since I had already committed one.

So it was just the next logical step that I went to a kegger. There, I met that other girl he had been with. He hadn't spoken to her since either. We became fast friends and gave him so much shit for being an asshole to *both* of us that he left in a hurry.

And that was that.

The whole thing really was all very matter of fact.

I wish I had known better than to try and use sex to keep a man. I wish that that experience had actually taught me that lesson. What I learned, unfortunately, from that lesson was that men (boys) want sex. And if you want a man, you have to give him sex. But you can do it on your own terms. But you have to do it.

I also wish that my friend, the one who had told me she lost her virginity, had included the part about how it was rape. She didn't tell me that until about six years later. I still want to punch that guy.

Has my attitude toward sex changed since then? Of course.

Has my attitude toward my mother? No.

Talk to your kids about sex! Openly! Honestly! Encourage them to wait but don't make it taboo! Teach them how to respect the opposite sex! Instill in them a healthy attitude towards sex!

I didn't have a horrible first time. But I could have. And I did have a long road of reprogramming my brain, relearning what I needed to know and think about sex.

Glitter

P IS FOR PLEASURE

Polly Priss

Acceptable outside, freaky inside. Hoping to one day merge the two and take over the world.

When I was five, I broke the star that sat upon the Christmas tree. I felt bad. I was angry with myself and wanted to be punished to help alleviate that guilt. My parents weren't around much, and even when home, they were not disciplinarians. So I sat myself in a corner. And I liked it. Age play has been in my pleasure pocket ever since.

For my seventh birthday I got a Cabbage Patch Kid and a package of real baby diapers for her. Everyone at the party laughed. They teased me, saying the diapers were for me. Well, there's an idea! I took them home and loved them. They smelled like powder. They crinkled softly. I was intrigued. I tucked them into my panties and used them. Afterwards they were warm and squishy. I masturbated. Then I snuck the used diapers to the trashcan and buried them, terrified of being caught.

I seem to have attached shame to sexual feelings from the very beginning.

My teenage years were full of kink, but not age play. Some kinks are hard to share, because they are rare, or less accepted. And high school is a fairly uncertain time as it is. I didn't share these parts of myself because they were too intimate. I hid these things away. Shame grew.

I graduated, moved out, married young, and had kids. I mentioned slight age play, like spanking, to my husband, but he wasn't into that at all, which furthered my shame. I avoided age play entirely during my early adult years. Perhaps I had enough diapers to worry about with my babies, but I also knew I wasn't with a supportive partner. I was certain my diaper fetish would go with me to the grave!

When I divorced and began dating an older man, I felt something awaken within me. I wanted to be little again. I was developing a new power, a desire to go after life. I wanted the things I'd always dreamed about to come true. My boyfriend and I had an organic D/s dynamic. Age play came quite naturally to us. I called him 'Daddy' from early on. He spanked me and teased me and I purred. But it took some time before I revealed my diaper fetish to him.

I prepared by writing about it on an anonymous LiveJournal, diving deep into my past, my needs, my reasons, my fears, my shame. I looked at it from all angles. Was I unloved as an infant? Potty trained too early? Why did I love the smell and the feel of diapers as an adult woman? Why did that get me off? What was wrong with me? I joined LiveJournal groups, and met other people who got off in diapers! I let them support me as I came to terms with my desires. I drew inspiration from these other journeys and I gained the confidence to go after what I wanted.

After months of journaling, I decided to let my boyfriend read it all. I was scared sick. But he was so amazing! He ordered diapers for me! Powdery-smelling crinkly ones! And thick white cotton ones! And pins! The first time we played with them I was an emotional wreck. I felt so bad about myself. Shame made my face hot, and tears rolled. For something that turned me on so much, my first time being diapered wasn't sexy at all! It was more of an intense therapy session that ended with pee running down my legs, forming a puddle at my feet as I sobbed! But we got through it!

The more we played, the less control shame had over me. It helped seeing how much my boyfriend enjoyed diapering me. I had built up these walls over my life, certain that something was wrong with me, embarrassed by sexual desires that were also deep emotional needs. I am still fighting with those feelings. In fact, just writing this piece has caused me some turmoil. It seems I'm still battling the shame that comes when seeking pleasure from outside the widely acceptable menu.

I may never be fully comfortable with my diaper fetish. Most of my diaper play is still in private, and not always due to shame. I know I can share it with my partner, but that doesn't mean I always want to. From the beginning, my diaper play was part of my masturbation ritual, and that is how I like it the most. I find pleasure holding it in until my bladder is dangerously full, then letting it go, just before I orgasm.

I am lucky to have an accepting and supportive partner, something I really worked for and went after. But it is also okay to embrace kinks on a private, personal level. It doesn't matter why I want this, why I like this, or when it began. What matters is that I'm living an authentic life and learning to embrace myself. I'm continually beating back the shame, replacing it with pleasure.

FIRE TRUCK!

Belle

I'm your average: customer service worker, married, mid-thirties, two kids and infertile.

I was never a whore in the classic sense of the word. Ex-boyfriends and ex-lovers were always my kryptonite. I met my first "boyfriend," 'C', online way before it was socially acceptable to do so. My mom let us go to the movies while she sat in the back. I was thirteen. Nothing happened then. My first school boyfriend was the popular guy. The class clown. I was fourteen, twenty-eight days away from being fifteen when I lost my virginity to him. A serious boyfriend followed and there was nothing too exciting sexually up until this point.

I always loved having a story. Being able to say

"yeah, I fucked him," or "yeah, I totally had sex while driving." I loved older guys, guys at least five years older than me. My girlfriends and I always talked openly about our conquests, there was even one summer we all had sex in the same room almost every night. I am proud to say that I took three men's virginities, that I'm aware of.

There wasn't an insane amount of men before I got married but I feel I had my share.

The one with the penis so small & the ego so big. This one got mad when we broke up so I called him at two a.m., woke him up and told him his dick was the smallest thing I had ever seen.

And it was.

The one who literally lasted ten seconds one time and should not count against my total. Amusingly, he knows my husband and I still run into him from time to time.

He really shouldn't count.

The guy my best friend was fucking with a fourteen-inch dick.

It was so big she made him take it out and show me.

It was *amazing*.

The first boyfriend who became a fuck buddy.

Someone to call on a lonely Friday night. He was the first man I was fucking but had no desire to date. He always wanted to cuddle after sex and I used to lie and leave my apartment and drive around the block so he would go home.

The boyfriend with the uncut dick I was afraid of and then realized how wonderful it was.

And how wonderful he wasn't.

The gay best friend who taught me how to give a really good blow job and how to have not painful anal sex.

The fuck buddy who was my first and only threesome. He fucked me doggie style in my best friend's closet while I blew his friend. Wonder why he never wanted to date me. :)

The year before I met my husband I had sex with four of my exes, going all the way back to the one who took my virginity. It was as if somehow I knew the next boyfriend was it and that this was my last opportunity.

I'm a faithful person. Now that I'm married and have been with my husband for over ten years it's no longer about the conquests but about how to make it interesting. We pride ourselves in unusual places. I gave him a hand job on an airplane in our seats with my father and brother seated behind us. In a fire truck. On the beach. On the hood of my car.

I often wonder what happens as we age and grow as a couple.

Will unusual places be enough?

Will porn and thongs and dildos be enough?

I can't imagine ever fucking or doing anything like that behind his back. I could however imagine it being done with his knowledge. With him watching? With me watching? I don't consider a hand job cheating, and I wouldn't be mad if he got one. I'm not sure if he ever would.

I look forward to our sexual future and I hope it's as exciting as I imagine it could be.

JUST CURIOUS

Krissy

I'm a curious southern girl stuck in Small Town rural Texas. I was born in 1989. That puts me at age twenty three. Fairly young but old enough that I'm just starting to get really comfortable with being open about my sexuality, even if things are a bit...confusing.

The lines of my sexual orientation are blurry at best. I've been married to a wonderful man for a couple of years now. I love him to death and the sex is absolutely amazing. But sometimes I really

46

feel like I'm missing out on something that could be equally amazing, something that could fulfill this need that's lurking around within me. Let's backtrack to my childhood.

I've always felt a lot of confusion when it comes to girls. It sounds so cliché, I know, but it's entirely true. At age five, I can remember thinking that my best friend was the prettiest girl I knew. At age seven, I remember having a crush on my female teacher. Things started to get murkier around age eight or nine. I was spending the night with a new, slightly older friend. She was about eleven, I think. Things were just like any other sleepover, until we crawled into bed for the night.

It's hard to remember exactly how things like that start, especially since it happened so long ago. Mainly I remember being in bed with the lights off and her saying something about kissing and how she really liked to do it. Before I knew it our lips were pressed together. I had never felt anything like it. It was sensational! Being in the dark, doing something I'd never done before, with someone I wasn't even sure I was allowed to be doing it with.

After a few seconds she pulled away and stared at me. It was about a minute before she spoke.

"Do you want to do it again?" she asked.

I nodded.

This time I was ready.

I only thought I was ready. She blew my mind even further on the second kiss. Our lips met, but this time she opened her mouth! I could feel her tongue trying to reach mine. I went with it. It was even more exhilarating than the one before. This felt so much more intimate, although I'm not sure I would've been able to describe that feeling back then. This time, I could feel exactly how soft her lips were. I could taste the lingering minty freshness of her toothpaste. Could feel her breathing heavily. I put my hand in her thick chestnut hair like I saw in the movies. It was so soft. I recall wishing it never had to end.

That was my first and only experience with kissing for a long time to come.

A few years went by and things were normal, mostly. I had crushes on boys and celebrities just like any other preteen girl. Boys invited me to dances, where we'd spin slowly on the floor and maybe hold hands. Afterwards I'd go spend the night with one of my girl friends. Nothing unusual ever really happened with many of them.

There was one friend that always wanted to shower together. She was cute, so I didn't turn her down. We never did anything, not even one little touch. Just washed up together, but it was very fun and exciting to see her like that. Sadly one of my many missed opportunities.

At age fifteen I got my first boyfriend and first real kiss from a boy. In that regard, I guess you could call me kind of a late bloomer. At least in comparison to all the rest of my friends. It wasn't that I didn't have anyone interested in me, I just wasn't very interested in any of them.

He was a nice boy. A bit punk rock, which is a type I still go for today, but very smart, respectful, and above all, hilarious. I liked him a lot, and we spent the first few weeks kissing like there was no tomorrow. Things were rolling right along, progressing both emotionally and physically. After hearing so many horror stories, I didn't want to get too physical without proof that we were pretty serious, relationship wise. Everything really got moving once he said he loved me.

The kissing was fun and it felt nice, but not as exciting as I remembered it to be. Lots of tongue and wetness and slurping sounds. Touching and being touched was infinitely more arousing. No one had ever touched me before. It was like a learning experience for my senses. Together we discovered that my breasts, especially my nipples, were very sensitive to being touched by hands that weren't my own. With him, I achieved my first orgasm that wasn't given to me by yours truly. I loved every bit of attention I was receiving. It felt good, and I was in love.

I also learned a lot about giving attention. His penis was the first I'd seen in real life. It seemed big in my hands, and was very smooth. I was a little disappointed though, because it didn't seem as erotic as I thought it would. It didn't excite me to play with it like it excited me to be played with. But I loved him, so I learned what to do and how he liked it anyways. Even though it didn't turn me on like I had hoped, I still felt a kind of satisfaction in giving him pleasure.

We moved on to oral sex soon, and I was unimpressed with both ends of it. I felt self-conscious when he was down there. What if it smelled weird? What if I tasted bad? It's really difficult to enjoy yourself when you're so worried about not being good enough. Giving wasn't much better. I wasn't sure what to do with my mouth. I gagged often.

We dated for two years. Things never did progress to penetration. We tried it once, but I wasn't ready. I was nervous. I wasn't in the mood. I wasn't even wet. He tried pushing into me. Slowly, but it hurt anyway. Thankfully he stopped when I asked him to. Looking back, I have mixed feelings about waiting. On the one hand, I wasn't truly ready for sex. On the other, we really did love each other, which is something I'm not sure I can say about the guy I did lose my virginity to.

I was eighteen, in my first semester of my freshman year of college, and still a virgin. I was making friends, going to parties and drinking lots of beer. One night my roommate and I were at a frat party. It was pretty laid back, just a bunch of guys and a couple of us girls sitting around a fire outside the house. A nice change from the big house parties and after-parties we were used to going to. After an hour or two and a few beers, the cute girl from my math class showed up. It turns out she was friends with a few of the same guys, we just didn't know it until she showed up at the party.

Looking around, there was nowhere for her to sit. All of the chairs and makeshift seats were already taken. She was across the fire from me, peering around, hoping for someone to get up. She noticed me. I waved hello and got a big smile in return. To my surprise, she came over and sat down on my lap. Having another girl sit on my lap wasn't too unusual for me, but normally it was someone I was already good friends with. We were just kind of acquaintances.

I remember her being very light. Lighter than I expected her to be. It didn't feel at all uncomfortable to have her there. After a few minutes we were talking and laughing it up and most of the guys had stopped staring at us. She picked up the giant purse she'd brought with her and pulled out a mostly empty bottle of Smirnoff vodka. The night was getting colder, and she seemed to nestle into me a little. It made my heart skip a beat for her to be so close to me. I wasn't sure, but it felt so much like she wanted to be there. I liked it.

By the end of the night I was very drunk, and I'd grown to like her a lot. We'd shared most of the vodka and several very steamy kisses by the fire. And right there in front of everyone, too! I have to admit, nobody really seemed to mind that sight, and I wasn't averse to letting it happen.

When she asked if I wanted to go back to her place, I didn't hesitate. Her behavior and the vodka had me riled up and I was ready for whatever was about to happen. We made the five minute drive in her 2007 Mustang back to her little efficiency apartment. Every second in that car felt like electricity between us. Was I really about to live out one of my longest running fantasies? Before I'd even had sex with a boy?! I was, and I was excited.

We pulled into her assigned parking spot and got out of the car. She unlocked the door and we practically fell inside kissing. We shut the door behind us, clothes dropping to the floor as we moved back to the bed. She removed my bra and hers and we were both down to our panties. Embarrassingly enough, I still had my socks on. It's one of those little details that I'm sure I'll never forget. Her soft, smooth, small hands felt like heaven against my skin.

She was beautiful to me, even with the lights off. Her shoulder length brown hair with its subtle highlights felt fluid and silky in my fingers. Big brown doe eyes opposite my blue ones, both filled with lust. The little bit of moonlight that was filtering in through the curtains made her skin look creamy and delicate.

At this point, I was still very drunk. I heard the door open. One of the frat boys was there. It seemed like she was expecting him, so I wasn't alarmed. In fact, I was intrigued. The night was taking yet another unexpected turn.

She motioned for him to come into bed with us. A tiny part of my brain was telling me that maybe losing my virginity in a threesome wasn't the best idea. The heat between my legs was telling me otherwise.

He came to me first, removing his clothes as he kissed me and moved us into a laying position. I'm not sure which of them removed my panties, but two sets of fingers found me. We spent a few minutes this way, kissing each other and them touching me. She told him to move aside, that she wanted me to herself for a few minutes. I wasn't sad about it. I liked her better. She was pretty and funny and her hands were softer and knew exactly where to touch.

I wish I could say that we continued into the night, but the alcohol got the best of me. My stomach was not having any more of this laying down business, even if the rest of me was burning to keep going. I ended up being sick and had to call another friend to come and get me. No virginities were lost that night.

That was my biggest and best experience with another girl to date. Looking back, I regret having had so much to drink. I often wonder what exactly would've happened if I had been able to stay. How would things be different today, if at all?

I ended up losing my virginity a couple of months later. It was with a guy I had started dating very shortly after the last incident. He had a bit of a reputation for sleeping around, but said that I was different. He said he wanted to treat me with care because I was a virgin. He didn't want to take that from me if it wasn't what I wanted. We thought we loved each other, so we did it.

I wish I could say it was memorable for all of the right reasons, but for the most part, it was one big let-down. It took us forever to get my roommate to leave, and then we realized that we didn't have a condom. A trip to the gas station was made. We got back and rushed to get started. It was over in less than five minutes. And it hurt. After the events and excitement of the last few months, I had been hoping for a much more enjoyable time. We dated for a while after that. Not one single time did he concern himself with my pleasure. In the following years, I'd have a few more sexual encounters, but nothing really worth mentioning.

Today, I'm married to a great guy that I've known my entire life. We go together like peanut butter and jelly. I enjoy being married, and I'm very happy, but I feel like I've missed out on experiencing what I desire. We've discussed it, and he is open to me experimenting if I can find the right girl who's up for the task. The one problem with that is that I'm not sure how to go about finding her.

First of all, I'm married. That's pretty off-putting for the majority of people. They see it as wrong. It's hard to explain that it's something my husband and I have agreed on in a way that they can understand and justify to themselves. It would be easier to pick some girl up at a bar, but I wouldn't want to be her drunken regret, for any reason.

Secondly, it's a lot more difficult than you might think to find a girl who is interested in a physical same sex relationship. Sure, a lot of girls my age will kiss other girls, but in my experience it's more of a 'party trick' for them. Not something they'd like to pursue further. I find that misleading, and trying to make my next move often ends up ruining what was, or what could have been, a good and lasting friendship.

Looking back, and while writing this, I've come to realize that my experiences with girls have been fueled by lust and physical attraction, while most of my encounters with men have been based on emotion. I'm not saying I could never form an emotional connection with another girl, but I will say that I don't know what this discovery says about myself. At times I'm still confused about where I stand sexually. Even though I've discussed it with my husband, it's hard to decide how I should go about figuring it out. Hopefully I will be able to make some decisions and find a girl who can help me in my quest for self-discovery. Until then, I'll keep fantasizing.

GAMES CHILDREN PLAY

Clara's BFF

Accountant living in the midwest with my husband, furbabies and son.

My family came to America when I was about six years old. I was immediately put into day care so my parents could work two jobs each to make a life for their family in the new county. I remember my first friend, Clara. She was also a child of newly arrived immigrants. We became instant friends, hanging out almost daily.

My new friend Clara's family had a nice family room in the basement where we could sit around and watch movies undisturbed. She preferred romantic chick flicks. I didn't. But she was the type of person who always got what she wanted.

By the time we were about eight, our games

evolved from playing romantic games with dolls, to acting out romantic situations or movies with revised plots. As I said before, her favorite movies were romances. We'd play knights and princesses or some adaptation of that, always with a damsel in distress, taking turns being the boy and being the girl. The knight would save the princess, woo her, and then they would fall into bed together. And the game would continue. We would always end up semi naked, touching each other in very inappropriate places. I guess I can consider that the first time I was fingered.

We never kissed. I guess she considered that outside the scope of the game. I never even really thought about any of it. I just did what she wanted, never thinking of how culturally 'wrong' it was. Let me clarify something, I have always been a sexual person, even before sex was a word that meant anything to me. Some people say they've never masturbated. I can remember masturbating even as a small child, in some of my earliest memories. It was always in bed at night, and even then I knew it was 'wrong' and I tried not to let my parents catch me. Back then it wasn't to orgasm (I didn't even know what an orgasm was), it just felt good. So I guess it would make sense that in my child's mind these games never seemed strange.

It got to the point that every time we hung out, which would be every weekend (as we got older our parents moved further apart from each other so

Glitter

soon weekends were the only times we could hang out), these were the only games we played. It was all we did. After a couple years I got tired of these games. I wanted to do something else. And as I got older I began to realize how 'wrong' these games were. Because Clara was used to getting her way, me telling her no didn't go over well. After a point we started to drift apart in our friendship until we stopped hanging out altogether.

Sex has never been a huge deal to me. I know that there are women who mistake sex and love. I was never one of those people. I lost my virginity on my sixteenth birthday, much earlier than most people I know. Granted it was with someone I was dating at the time, but it was more because he wanted to and I just didn't care enough to argue with him. It wasn't at all that I was madly in love with him and it meant something special thing to me. There were no flowers and dim lighting. It was more like 'this hurts like a bitch so let's just get it over with.'

In college I had many friends with benefits. Don't get me wrong, I wasn't super promiscuous. I kept the same 'friends' for long stretches of time. I still preferred to play it safe and not screw too many people for fear of contracting diseases, but I never had issues with keeping just the friends with benefits status. I never wanted a relationship from someone just because we'd drunk dial each other in the middle of the night.

I often wonder if my casual stance on sex had to do

with those early childhood games. To be honest I have thought of those early years a lot, especially during my more promiscuous times. They say that a person's childhood shapes their adult years. I wonder sometimes what kind of impact it had on me. Sometimes I'm grateful for it since it made anything sexual a non-traumatic experience for me, something I was prepared for. I don't feel mentally broken. I'm pretty happy with the person I've become. Would I want the same experience for my children? No. It still feels, for lack of a better word, 'icky'. But for me it seemed to work.

DEAREST BOB

Meg

I live in an extremely small, conservative town where everyone knows your name. I live here with my dog where I make my living as a writer/photographer/office worker. I first discovered the wonderful world of boys (and girls) in the early 1990s where Eddie Vedder and Kurt Cobain infiltrated my dreams.

I was twenty-two when we met.

I was introduced to Bob at a party by my friend B.

She had been acquainted with him for years and thought it was time she introduced the two of us.

I was nervous.

I didn't have much experience with dating and when it came to sex, I had absolutely no experience. I spent my teenage and college years watching friends date and swap boyfriends/girlfriends like baseball cards. I grew up in a small town where everyone knows everyone and spent kindergarten through senior year of high school with the same group of kids. I grew up being told by my grandmother that if I was just a little prettier, because I'll never be beautiful, and lost some weight, then maybe a boy would ask me out on a date. I was taught that even though some of my friends were having sex, good girls didn't have sex. That was something you only did with your husband. On top of that, I was a fat girl and no one wanted to date, let along fuck fat girls. Sure there had been boyfriends. There were a lot of make-out sessions, but nothing beyond that and nothing they wanted to talk about.

B assured me that he wouldn't care. He didn't have a type. He loved all women: big, small, fat, skinny, tall, short, it didn't matter, he loved them all, knew what they needed and knew how to treat them right.

I trusted B and knew she wouldn't steer me wrong. So I took him home after the party. I had butterflies in my stomach the entire ride to my apartment. I didn't know what to expect but was assured he would take care of me. I would be fine. That I would like it.

Once at my apartment we went straight to the bedroom. No idle chit chat. No unnecessary pleasantries. It was just right down to business. I don't think I've ever stripped out of my clothes as fast as I did that night.

We quickly settled into an easy rhythm. He took some getting used to but once I relaxed I was toast, totally giving in to his moves.

We started slow, with long easy strokes before gradually increasing pressure, speed, changing positions. First on my back until I relaxed, then to my knees to even deeper penetration. And what he did with my clit, I never wanted him to stop.

I had no idea it could feel this way. I had tried bringing myself to orgasm plenty of times before but had never quite gotten there. I'd always been close, but never managed to tip myself over the edge.

But with Bob – sweet, sweet Bob – it didn't take long. The first orgasm came too quickly. So quickly I didn't know what was happening. I tried to hold it off, but couldn't stop it no matter how hard I tried. It left me shaking and breathless but I wanted more.

The second came on slower. It was less frantic, more controlled. Starting at my toes, engulfing me like a warm blanket before a wave of pleasure washed over me. It was one of the most satisfying feelings I had ever had. Afterwards I sank contentedly back into my bed.

The first night with Bob was the first of many. Together he and I discovered what I liked and what I didn't like. How much pressure I liked and where. He's been there when I've needed a stress reliever after work when boyfriends haven't quite been able to get me to where I needed to be.

On the few occasions boyfriends have been open to using toys, he was able to join in on the fun.

If someone would have told me I would have lost my virginity to a vibrator, I would have been mortified. I would have told them they were crazy. There was no way I would ever use a toy especially for something as important as that! But I did, loved everything about it and wouldn't trade that in for anything.

INVISIBLE BISEXUAL

Delilah Night

Delilah Night is an American living in Singapore with her husband and young children. With unlimited time and money, she would become either a sexologist or a pastry chef. She invites you to visit her website, DelilahNight.com.

To the casual observer, I would appear straight.

I'm married to a person of the opposite sex, and we have two daughters.

I'm not straight. I'm an invisible bisexual.

Growing up in a small rural town, I was taught to treat everyone the same. Yet my family expressed disgust at the idea of two men kissing in public. I would hear things like "why can't they just keep it in the bedroom?" It's better than "they're evil and going to hell," I suppose, but not by much.

I learned that a relationship with another person of my sex was wrong, dirty, and something I should keep secret. I thought that there were only two possibilities: that I would be attracted to males or to females. The idea that you could be sexually attracted to both sexes was completely foreign.

As I approached middle school, my sexuality began to blossom.

When I stole my mom's bodice rippers, I was a bit grossed out by the descriptions of the hero's turgid manhood (and had never seen a penis), so I skipped those parts and focused instead on the heaving breasts of the heroine.

I found a discarded men's magazine at the campground across the street from our trailer and became fascinated with one of the photos: a naked woman, legs spread, fingers holding her labia open, displaying her clit (although I didn't have any of those words, either. I knew 'vagina', but we mostly called it "down there"). I knew I couldn't take the magazine home, so I hid it in some bushes and went back to visit it daily until a night of rain destroyed it.

Confusing the issue was the fact that I was supposed to like boys. The boys in my fifth grade class were immature morons. Who would want to kiss them?

Relief, along with attraction, flooded my body when *Star Trek: The Next Generation* spawned my first real crush in 1990: Wil Wheaton. Case closed: I was straight, and I was grateful.

In high school, I began experimenting with boys. I liked kissing boys. I liked the tangible proof of their arousal when 'hanging out' turned into making out. I liked it when they slid their hands under my shirt. Those 'turgid manhoods' of the bodice rippers were no longer repulsive.

I would think about girls, but when those thoughts turned sexual I told myself that what I felt was envy or aspiration. That I wanted to be like them, not be with them. It's not like I was a lesbian – I liked making out with boys – so I was straight.

A lesbian wouldn't enjoy making out with boys. I couldn't picture any other explanation.

When I became sexually active, I chose male partners.

In college, I constructed a new explanation for my confusion without modifying my identity as a straight woman: *Society teaches us that women are sexually desirable. It's only normal that I should find women attractive. It's society's fault, not mine.*

I told myself that when I would wake up from a dream involving a woman. When I'd masturbate and the person I was thinking about suddenly became a woman. Even finding my panties and cunt wet with arousal after hanging out with a woman I liked (as a friend) didn't change my identity as a straight woman.

I shared my theory about society and female attraction with my best friend. She agreed with me (which meant I was right). I was straight and it was society's fault I was attracted to other women. It wasn't a real thing, just the by-product of social conditioning.

My best friend and I continued to blame society for every girl we thought of as sexy.

We even used my theory to justify experimenting. Just to see what it would be like. Because society had taught us that we should want to experience the difference between men and women's lips. We ended up on my dorm bed. Lipstick smeared, bras abandoned, fingers sliding into panties. Afterward we went out to a night club and made a point of dirty dancing with men because, dammit, we were STRAIGHT.

It was awkward when she decided that our make-out session had satisfied her curiosity. That maybe at some later time she might do it again, but for now it was all penis all the time. I didn't feel the same.

Even though by that point I had gay friends and had divorced myself of the prejudices of my upbringing, I just couldn't wrap my head around my own sexuality. Had I been attracted solely to women, I could have understood that. Wanting both men and women made me feel guilty. Why couldn't I just pick?

This is the heart of one of the most harmful and common tropes of bisexuality: that we are greedy, slutty fence sitters who are unwilling to limit ourselves to partners of one sex. I should know how harmful it is, it's the argument with which I berated myself.

Admitting that I sought counseling from my college's therapists is somewhat embarrassing, but

I needed to talk to someone, to say things aloud that I'd kept quiet for a long time, and they provided a safe environment. Within a few months of that make out session, I came out to someone for the first time. My friends accepted me. My mom decided it was a phase I'd soon be over, just as I'd gotten over my goth phase, and rolled her eyes.

While reaching the conclusion that I was bi was a challenge, once I made peace with it, I was quite happy to define myself as bisexual.

I spent the rest of my early and mid-twenties dating and fucking my way through a swath of partners. I hooked up at bars with men and women. I did online dating (although only with guys, since there was no bisexual box to check). I spent hours chat-fucking men and women on instant messenger. I was young enough to enjoy wallowing in the drama of my various relationships. I wasn't terribly preoccupied with activism or what labels people wanted to apply to me. I just liked sex.

The one exception to this easy dismissal of labels happened when I was living in New York City. I was really horny and wanted to hook up with a girl that night, so I went to a lesbian bar I'd found in the LGBT section of *Time Out* magazine. Butterflies flitted nervously in my stomach as I entered. What if they could tell I liked fucking guys, too? Would they think I was just one of those 'lesbian until graduation' types? Was I a total phony? I ended up sitting at the bar, only making eye contact with my amaretto sour. I never went back.

When I was twenty-seven I fell in love with a man, and we married. It was around this age that I started to care about activism (spurred by the gay marriage battle in my home state). I'd long considered myself part of the gay community as an ally but now I began to define myself as a member of the community. I wanted to speak out, to be a visible member of the community.

It's ironic, really, that just as I decided to become visible as a member of the queer community, everyone else had officially declared me to be straight. After all, I had 'picked'. I was a woman who had married a man. Woman + man = straight. I'm sure that people had assumed I was straight every time I'd had a boyfriend, but I'd never cared about it before.

I'm not straight.

When I tried to be out as bisexual, but married to a man, it often led to intrusive questions like...

"So if your husband's a guy, how do you handle being attracted to women?"

"Do you cheat on him with women?"

"But you really *prefer* men, right? I mean, you married one..."

Married bisexuals (or bisexuals in committed relationships) occupy a barren territory. We are seen to have picked our team (straight or gay), and should just shut up. When we show up with our families at Pride events, we are welcomed as allies, not as members of the community.

While we've come a long way in recognizing gays and lesbians, bisexuals have long been ostracized by the gay community. We are a fringe group, and we don't fit neatly into a box. The default assumption is that our sexuality reflects the sex of our partner, and we are treated accordingly: straight or gay.

We end up invisible.

What does bisexual pride look like? What does bisexual equality mean? That there isn't an easy answer, or perhaps even an answer at all beyond "accept that sexuality is a fluid continuum and not a binary," makes our place in the fight for acceptance messy at best.

I will absolutely grant that in many ways, we bisexuals in opposite sex relationships have the easiest road when compared to the rest of the LGBT community. We can get married in all fifty states. We don't have to worry about our children's schools accepting our families as families. No one is arguing that we are not the gender we know ourselves to be.

That doesn't mean that it's easy to be an invisible bisexual.

I can stand right in front of you and you'll never see me. Or believe I exist. You'll think I went through a phase that I'm now over. Or you'll want sordid details of my sex life to justify my assertion that I am, in fact, bisexual.

There's no secret bisexual society that I'm required to report to. There is not a quota of women I have to fuck each year to qualify as bisexual. No one is going to knock on my door and order me to turn in a membership card if I don't masturbate equally to men and women.

You see me with my husband and my kids, but you don't really see me.

THE CELIBATE SLUT

Jess

I am a mental health professional, pastry chef, ex-art major, crazy cat lady, fat model, fiery advocate, and total pain in the ass. You can read more about me on my web site TheMilitantBaker.com.

I'm a twenty-six-year-old professional with a grown up career and other big kid responsibilities, but five years ago I was an ambitious and talented professional drunk. This consequentially landed me the title of 'slut' but I like to think about myself as being "a lady of the evening making up for lost time."

I grew up strictly religious, scared of my body, never knowing quite fully about my anatomy, and convinced that someday I would find Prince Charming and we would get married, ride to a castle and hug all night. Fast forward to a party with what my Mom called the "wrong crowd" when I was nearly twenty-one, where after I finished my very first bottle of Jack Daniels I found myself in a hammock with a sexy bar bouncer receiving my first kiss. Twenty years old and I didn't have the foggiest idea about how you are supposed to kiss. I think I ended up sucking a lot of hollow air. Luckily we were both drunk enough to not care and continued macking all night.

Shitfaced, I went to bed and he asked if he could sleep in my room as well. Any other person on the planet would have known what this actually meant, but I really just thought we would crash on the floor and get a good night's sleep. But, instead I was date raped. For years I thought it was my fault, and held on to the massive amount of guilt that accumulated. I remember calling a friend, sobbing into the phone about how confused I was at what to do next, I had heard about Planned Parenthood but that was the extent. She asked me if he "came in" me and I didn't know what that meant so I said yes to save myself from seeming even more inexperienced. It was only years later that I realized that I was simply a young naive girl who didn't know anything about anything and was taken advantage of by someone who knew goddamn well what he was doing. This was a hard realization, but now that I look back it explains perfectly how the next few years came about.

Now, don't get me wrong, the whirlwind of consensual sex was a riot after that. I became the talk of the town while adoring every rumor. I spent every night in a club or bar, dancing my ass off and having a great time. And every night I had a new partner usually exploring anything and everything under the sun. Er, moon. I couldn't tell you the names of most of them and some memories are fuzzy but I had a hell of a good time. Public sex under the staircase across the street, in alleys, cars, random people's beds and couches, bathtubs, pool tables... phenomenal. Alcohol loosened me up and quickly turned this virgin into a kick-ass tramp.

My first real relationship was a sidewalk meeting one drunken 4th of July night with a carney from the circus. Within ten minutes of meeting we were in a cab on the way to my house and thus started a three-year stint with toxic love and sexual deviation. I learned about everything with the carney, and there was no shame. We fingered each other at the top of the Capitol building in DC. We had riotous sex in a circus train with paper-thin walls and an old chef masturbating next door. We found a mutual love of S&M and bondage and sexted graphic wet dreams all day long, It was excessive, but it was also the basis for the relationship and so it fueled us and we ran with it.

After the devastating but necessary end of that clusterfuck, I reveled in the single life again. I placed personal ads on Craigslist and each time I did, my inbox would fill with hundreds of responses. I had a 'date' every night and would meet them at my favorite bar which was a five minute walk from my house. This worked perfectly as the bouncers were close friends, the beer was cheap, and it took less than an hour for me to deem them safe and get their eager bodies into my bed. It was odd for me to go without sex for more than a couple of days.

Through this though, I met my current long-term boyfriend who was different than the rest. I love him dearly and the sex was good...but only for four months.

We've now been together for two years and within the last year and a half we have had sex once. This devastated me for more than a year, leaving me in tears every night sure that it was because I was awful in bed or my body wasn't adequate. We eventually learned however, that because of childhood trauma he wasn't able to connect on a physical level after a serious emotional connection was made. I still feel cheated, even today, but we are both seeking therapy and I'm sure that eventually we will get back into the swing of vanilla sex. I'm okay with once-in-a-while plain ol' sex, and I have my debauched past to thank for that. I've been there, done that, and while it's hard, my current boyfriend is worth the wait. And that night when I do get laid, well, that will probably seem like the best sex of my life.

KINKY GIRL

Lucky Girl

I'm a Silicon Valley marketing person with an MBA who came of age in the 1990s.

I've been kinky as long as I can remember.

In my professional life I'm a very ambitious, smart, take-charge person. In my sexual life, I want to be dominated, bound, controlled and used.

In kindergarten, I would play tie-up games with my friends. It wasn't sexual, in a post-pubescence sort of way that it later became, but I liked it. I preferred to be tied up, but would dutifully switch off as needed to keep my friends interested in the game. I have no idea what gave me the idea in the first place.

I was an advanced reader, and in junior high I started going through my parents' bookshelves and found all sorts of pulpy historical fiction. I specifically remember a book about Anne Bonney, the pirate, and a scene where she was tied to the bed and teased. In junior high, I had a friend who would come over for sleepovers, and we'd come up with all sorts of stories that involved us being tied up and helpless.

I masturbated a lot as a teenager. At one point I tried to see how many times I could come in a row. I think I got to seven before I became tired out. My reading material was still limited largely to romance novels and pulpy historical fiction, and it turns out there's plenty of (gently) kinky sex in them, but at some point I picked up the A. N. Roquelaure *Beauty* books. Not sure how I heard about them. My mom at some point looked at the books when I was buying them and made some negative comment. Nowadays my mom brings up

Fifty Shades of Grey over lunch conversation.

I didn't date in high school (I was young), and really looked forward to college.

My first boyfriend in college – first semester of freshman year – was also my first sexual partner. Unfortunately, he laughed when I told him I wanted to be tied up. A few years later, when he was dating a friend of mine, I noticed handcuffs by his bed. He apologized for laughing at me. The first time I had sex wasn't particular enjoyable, in fact I think it took two or three tries before we really 'had sex' because it hurt. We're still friends.

My second and third boyfriends weren't kinky, not as far as I know, but at that point I was kinda scared off of telling people. I was in college in the early 1990s, when Usenet was active, and I spent a lot of time reading alt.sex.bondage and alt.sex.bondage.stories. I still have quite a collection saved from those days! So even though my relationships weren't kinky, my fantasy life certainly was!

Then I started dating a guy who was kinky. Unfortunately he was also a controlling, abusive asshole, though it took me too long to figure that out and even longer to do something about it. We starting dating the spring semester of my sophomore year, then through the summer, then we moved in together for junior year. We went to play parties and did some relatively soft public scenes (spanking or whipping). I learned a lot, mostly from reading alt.sex.bondage.

The summer after junior year I had an internship in a different city – at that point I knew I wanted out of the relationship, but since we lived together I hadn't managed to extricate myself. I had met someone at the end of my junior year who I enjoyed spending time with, and he and I traded a lot of email over the summer I was away. When I got back from the summer, I told my boyfriend (we shall refer to him as the evil ex) that I wanted to break up, and he hit me and dragged me by the hair, and coerced me into having sex with him; kinky sex, at that. Midway through I freaked out, and he hit me, which cut my lip and bruised my face. It's the only time in my life I thought I might die. But I didn't.

Soon after, I started dating the guy I met at the end of my junior year. He was kinky, but really in his heart wanted to be dominated. He was willing to dominate me, and enjoyed it, but wanted me to switch. And I did, but it wasn't a turn-on. In fact, it was something of a turnoff. It made him seem weak to me, and since my kink is about wanting to be dominated and controlled, that didn't play very well together. But coming off the abusive relationship, it worked for a long time.

Eventually I met the man I married, who is masculine, has a strong personality, is incredibly attractive, loves me and takes care of me. We had an immediate connection and at some point I told him I had a secret I needed to tell him. I admitted I was kinky, and that sexually I was submissive, and was delighted to find that he was compatibly kinky. We have vanilla sex, but nearly always laced with at least kinky conversation, and we also have extremely non-vanilla sex with toys and bondage and play and extra fabulous orgasms.

When I masturbate, it's always to fantasies that involve bondage and submission. I'm not particularly a masochist: it's the submitting that turns me on, more than the pain. I'm not into humiliation; feeling awkward or embarrassed just doesn't makes me feel sexy.

I feel incredibly lucky to have a partner who's so sexually compatible with me. I realized it's really important to me that I balance my public persona's Type A personality by being able to submit and give up control to someone else in the bedroom. It works really well for us.

HIDING IN PLAIN SIGHT

Nikkiana

Nikkiana lives in NYC with her sound engineer boyfriend, her magician roommate and her cat who can open the refrigerator. You can read her PG-13 adventures at AuthenticExperience.org.

"I was at a slumber party last night and my friend woke me up by touching my boobs and kissing me," she confessed, "and I liked it!"

In that moment, I suddenly understood the meaning of arousal. My mind raced with the possibilities.

"I wish something like that would happen to me at a slumber party," I lamented.

I was an awkward thirteen-year-old who over the past two years had developed a habit of sneaking into my parents' bedroom and reading their porno mags every time they left the house.

She was a nameless faceless girl on the internet that I had exactly two conversations with. She went by the moniker of "Hotpants" and she claimed she was eleven years old, and at the very least she typed like one. I suppose the reality might have been that she was really a forty-year-old inner tube salesman from Ohio, but I took her on face value.

Hotpants, with her confession of a slumber party fondling from a girl friend, had just induced the realization that I had a very strong desire to have the same thing happen to me. I found myself sitting in class sizing up the girls in the room. They fell into two categories, incredibly boy crazy or completely oblivious. No one seemed to be an obvious candidate for a slumber party make-out session.

I combed the internet looking for advice on how to tell if a girl would be willing to make out with you but tripped over the reality that same sex relations had an inherit social risk to them. Proposition the wrong girl, or hell, just admit the truth to the wrong person, and then be the butt of a reputation-smearing campaign. I was already having trouble making friends, I didn't need to do something that could make me a social pariah.

I kept my desires to myself, only voicing them to random strangers that I met on AOL chat rooms who claimed to be my age but probably weren't.

As the years progressed, I grew more and more socially withdrawn among my own gender. My disinterest in clothes and makeup combined with the fact that I couldn't sit in a group of girls without having fantasies of a lesbian group sex porn breaking out caused me to feel even more awkward than I already was, and I was terrified of becoming close friends with a girl because I knew that inevitably I was going to start crushing and want to get them into bed.

I fell into a group of social outcasts, a group of nerdy kids that was predominantly male and heavily Christian. Not only was being remotely not straight not cool, but so was the idea of sex altogether.

I wasn't entirely sold on the abstinence logic. I'd spent my early teens eating up Scarleteen.com and had internalized some degree of sex-positivity despite my anxieties about social acceptability, and despite the fact that my friends seemed to think abstinence was the only way. I thought differently.

I lost my virginity at sixteen to the first guy that offered. A fourteen-year-old long-haired Wiccan boy with an alcoholic mom who would ground him for looking at the dog the wrong way, who mostly hid out at his best friend's house down the street. He was my boyfriend for a whole month and it cost me my social circle for about four months as my friends stopped speaking to me because I dared to date someone.

At seventeen, desperate to fit in further with my friend circle I professed belief in God and started attending church with my friends. Despite some desire to be a 'good girl' who did things 'the right way', the new commitment caused me to start living a dual life.

I dated people and slept around, but I kept things hush-hush. I fooled around with people who were outside of my friend circle or at very least had the good sense to keep their mouths shut. I didn't make commitments and thus didn't remain monogamous to anyone.

When I started dating the man who eventually became my ex-husband not long after I began college, I finally decided I'd had enough with keeping my actions secret and went public with the fact that he was indeed my boyfriend. I started hemorrhaging friends, but at that point I had grown weary of the manipulation and was beginning to realize that these people were not really my friends.

However, I was still heavily under the spell of the church and I traded the manipulative group of friends of my teenage years for some equally manipulative adults who, in retrospect, seemed oddly interested in our sex life and in the name of Christ were trying to convince us that either we ought to get married or break up.

This continued until the pastor of the church decided to voice his distaste for my blogging habit and we decided that we didn't need a church that felt the need to criticize our every move anymore. No longer bound by the rules or criticism of the church, we were suddenly free to experiment...and we did.

Except for now I found myself in a position that I didn't really want to be in.

My ex had a strong desire for threesomes and group sex, and while I wasn't against the idea, I wasn't for it either. It was something I wanted to approach cautiously. He made the argument that this was probably the only way I'd ever end up in bed with a girl. One day, he found a girl he thought would be a good candidate and arranged a date for the three of us. She was nice, but I wasn't attracted to her.

He proceeded to drive us around to different bars and get us drunk, then suggested a threesome on the drive home. Despite the fact that I wanted to say no, the thought that I'd never otherwise sleep with a girl pervaded me and I said yes with the stipulation that there would be no penetration between them, a boundary that ended up violated within the first three minutes of the act.

The event was bittersweet. On the one hand, the sex was good. On the other, I hadn't really wanted to do this in the first place and I had a requested boundary violated. I focused on the positive and bottled up the negative. I was so conflicted that I couldn't find my own voice on the issue.

A few months later, we decided it might be nice to move in together, so we decided to get engaged and he moved in with me at my parents' house. Our sex life tanked, but I blamed it on the buzzkill of having a bedroom over the room where my parents watched TV. I was in denial that the real issue was we couldn't have sex without him bringing up how he wanted to fuck the girl from the threesome again.

We got married. We moved into our own apartment. We fought continuously over sex. He never wanted to have it, despite the fact that he would bog down our internet connection downloading porn. Despite not having moral issues with porn, I found myself feeling like I was being cheated somehow. Whenever we did have sex, he kept bringing up how he wanted to fuck the girl from the threesome again. Some days, I'd find myself screaming at him because of how undesired I felt. Other days, I just internalized it: figuring out a way to get off on being so undesirable that your own husband can't have sex with you without thinking of someone else.

Upon the suggestion of a friend, we tried opening our marriage. It wasn't a good decision: if you don't have a solid marriage to begin with, introducing other people doesn't do anything but introduce drama. But, briefly, we were happier. He wasn't feeling pressured for sex, and I was finding people to sleep with who were, quite frankly, far superior lovers. But it was unequal: I had a far easier time finding external lovers, and on the rare occasion that he actually did, I raged and scared them off.

Then we moved to New York City and our

relationship tanked into an irreparable state. He hated the city and refused to work. I developed a drinking problem and felt further under appreciated. One year in the Big Apple and I finally found my voice to say that this was not what I wanted, that I was tired of being treated like shit. I was tired of trying to save something that never was meant to be.

Not saying I was innocent either, but I finally had found my voice. I had finally figured out how to say what I wanted.

I met my current partner five days after my ex had moved back to whence he came. Our relationship has been a constant exercise in being honest about what we want, both in the bedroom and out of life. He constantly reminds me of how beautiful I am, and I consistently remind him how lucky I am to have him. Things aren't perfect, but we try our best to work through our problems, even the ones that aren't easy.

The journey is far from over. I'm glad it's just begun.

THE LEARNING CURVE OF
CRIPPLED SEX

Jenn

Jenn is a 20-something writer and wife who rocks harder than she rolls, sharing her stories about marriage, infertility, and life as a physically handicapped woman in the (not always so) accessible world on her blog, CrippledGirl.com.

If I wrote out a scene from my sex life, it would probably sound like an assault:

His breath was heavy as he hovered over me, using his rough hands to pull the clothes off my motionless body. Grabbing the back of my knees, he dragged me across the sheets towards the center of the bed. He put me exactly where he wanted me; I just laid there.

But it's not a horrific rape flashback or even some raunchy role play. It's just an average Tuesday night quickie, with my husband getting me into position for sex because I don't have the strength to move my body on my own.

Having a progressive, degenerative muscular disease has taken me from a wobbly-walking teenager to a fully wheelchair-bound, twenty-six-year-old woman. Although my disability has been challenging at times, the wheelchair certainly hasn't killed my libido. It may have even increased it, considering my sexuality is sometimes the only aspect of my body over which I have full control.

Adjusting sex to the physical limitations of my body definitely isn't always an easy thing. I'd be a liar if I said I was totally comfortable in my own skin or confident in my skill. I worry about how my lack of movement will impact my marriage almost every day.

Is he happy with our sex life? Is he frustrated at having to do all the work? Is he bored? Will he get bored and look for someone who can do the things I can't?

But by far, the worst fear comes from the worry that the stigma of abandoning his handicapped spouse will guilt him into staying, even if he truly isn't happy.

Since my condition is progressive, there are things I used to be able to do that I can't anymore. It also means that in five or ten years, I may not be able to do half of what I can do now. That fact is more than worry – it terrifies me. Will he still get a thrill of taking my clothes off when he has to help me put them on every morning? Will he still see the curves of my shape, and not just the cold, boxy, metal wheelchair?

My husband thinks I'm crazy for worrying about all this; and most days he's probably right. I really couldn't ask for a more devoted guy, who has been supportive and dedicated to every single minute of this learning curve, as we try to figure out how the hell to make 'crippled sex' work for the both of us.

When you get down to the core of it, our learning curve isn't really any different than any other couple's process of trial-and-error. We've had to explore and adapt to each other, figure out the sensations, places, and positions that are successful and rule out what doesn't work. The mobility issue just means we experiment on a different scale. Sometimes it's normal things, like placement of pillows and "my leg doesn't move that way, buddy," and other times we're discussing how a Hoyer lift or the angle tilt/recline feature on my wheelchair could work for bumpin' uglies.

Like all things in life, there are disguised blessings, beyond the ability to joke about manipulating medical equipment for sex. We've learned to laugh when something goes wrong, but more importantly, how to talk to each other to make it better. When your body doesn't move, you learn in a hurry just how important it is to vocalize what you need want and need.

In that sense, maybe everyone needs to have a little crippled sex.

THE OTHERS

Sweet Cheeks

Just a simple southern housewife with a naughty side.

On the surface I'm a conservative, minivan-driving housewife who's been happily married to her high school sweetheart for fourteen years. In reality, I'm proof that it really is "always the quiet ones."

My husband was my first, but by no means my last. How is that possible since we've been together since I was sixteen? During the latter part of college he decided that I should be with at least one other person before we got married in the next few years. The (first) other person? One of his best friends with whom who I'd shared obvious sexual tension for years. I'm not sure when the tension started, I just remember being attracted to him shortly after meeting him. He was one of those guys who knows exactly how to smile, look at, and talk to girls in a way that makes them melt. Often he'd openly flirt with me right in front of my boyfriend. One night he came to my boyfriend's apartment and had a movie for us to watch: "*Threesome*! I have never felt so much sexual tension. I was nineteen, terribly inexperienced, and very shy, so there was no way I was making a move or even letting on how much I wanted him.

Sometime in the next year he got a Prince Albert and afterwards felt the need to pull it out frequently just to make me blush. Finally after several years of flirting my boyfriend decided his friend and I should have sex. I never knew or wanted to know what their conversation arranging this entailed. It was a Saturday afternoon and my boyfriend left for the afternoon and left us alone, making it clear we should have fun. We did. We then hooked up on a few other occasions before he moved four hours away.

After not seeing him for over two years he moved back and needed a place to stay so my boyfriend let him stay there. The day he got in to town my boyfriend was gone, having to entertain some people from work who'd come to visit, so I was there to let him in. From the moment he arrived it was clear the sexual attraction was to pick up right where we left off. After flirting all afternoon he finally kissed me. He'd decided that we shouldn't have sex since he was living there. That didn't stop him from getting me off almost daily for the next few months. He ended up moving again but would return in a couple of months when my boyfriend and I got married.

Because of the way we'd left things it just made sense that we'd somehow hook up when he was here for the wedding. After the wedding we came back to our house as we weren't leaving town until the next day. He was staying there too. There were lots of drinks so I'm not clear how it came about but I think we'd gone to bed and my new husband went and asked him to join us. This was all new territory for all of us. I made out with him while my husband fondled me. My husband then fucked me while he watched me suck his friend's dick. It was the hottest thing he'd ever seen. Sadly, I never got off that night. I'm not sure why. Nerves, maybe? One of the ironies of my 'wedding night' being a threesome? My mom had bought me a white sequined nightgown, complete with bed jacket that she thought was perfect for a bride on her wedding night.

My boyfriend/fiancé's friend wasn't my only indiscretion. During grad school I ran into an old high school crush who happened to be working at the copy center near campus. He was fascinated by my feminist theory coursework and eager to get together to talk about books (yeah, I think we both knew that was BS). He called me late that night and we talked a while and at some point he told me he gave a great vulva massage (I couldn't make that up if I tried). We got together the following night and talking led to him giving me a foot massage (he admitted to a foot fetish), which led to massaging everywhere, which quickly led to making out in our underwear. This night was and still is the most turned on I've ever been. He slid his hand down my panties, barely touching me, and I immediately came. It was late and I went home soon afterward. I was dying to fuck him but being a good southern girl I felt that would be slutty.

He was one of those artsy creative types who are very attentive sexually. We got together pretty regularly for a while over the summer before I got married (yes, I was also fooling around with my fiancé's friend at the same time). My fiancé was extremely turned on by the thought of me being with someone else so on nights I'd go see my high school crush I'd then go to his house because he loved to fuck me knowing I was so wet because of what someone else had done. I didn't enjoy that part. I liked pleasing him but I felt that what I was doing with anyone else was mine to be enjoyed by only me. Retelling what I'd done earlier with someone else just made me feel dirty and whore-ish.

This pattern would carry over into the first two years of our marriage. We'd agreed at the time that we both wanted to be with other people in addition to each other. I went on to have a fling with another creative (great in bed) type and later a boring guy with the smallest dick I've experienced. I didn't like being with other people and sharing it with him. I went on to have a few other flings and keep them to myself but none of them were satisfying for long, I only felt dirty and often regretted getting married. I went on to gain & lose weight, become overall less sexual, and leave that life behind. Even up until a few years ago my husband would ask me to tell him stories from back then while we were having sex. It ruined sex for me and after being told numerous times how dirty it made me feel he stopped asking for the stories.

These days our sex life (or rather lack thereof thanks to parenting a small child) is just us, as 'vanilla' as can be.

THE FEAR

Lexie

I'm a dog walker by day, and a sexual deviant by night, although I've worn many different hats throughout the years. I live with my girlfriend of just over two years. I'm still trying to work out the sexual hiccups that come with being with someone faithfully for this long.

I came of age when I was eleven or twelve, about fifteen years ago. I remember being horrified when I had to tell my mom why I was late for the bus. I spent the entire day bleeding at school, wanting to crawl into a hole and die. That night I made her swear not to tell anyone. The next Christmas, I got a kaboodle filled with pads. Thanks, Mom. Four years later I lost my virginity and haven't stopped since.

I can't tell you much about the first time I was with a woman, I was swept up in a blizzard of booze and thrown against a bathroom countertop. Shampoo and hair products rolling to the ground, my mind hazed over and the next day I was barely able to remember the night before. The only thing lingering and making it real was the slight soreness between my legs. Not to mention the recurring phrase "You have a beautiful pussy" playing on repeat in my head, in her voice.

I had this fear inside my chest. The kind of fear that would tighten and cause my pale skin to turn seven different shades of red if ever confronted with it. That fear? Women. More specifically, women that were gay.

It was the end of a toxic relationship, the culmination of four years of hell. I moved out of the apartment with barely any notice and left my then ex-boyfriend to deal with the shambles. I was free! With the end of any romantic entanglement, I was left to sort out my self-esteem and my sex drive that was now in shambles.

My new roommate was an openly gay woman, about eight years my senior, that I knew through work. I wasn't attracted to her, but looked up to her strong attitude towards her sexuality. I needed to get that back in my life. I took a deep breath and told her to give her friend my number.

That previous Christmas I had met one of her best friends at our work's Christmas party. I was there with my now ex, but the instant I met her my chest tightened and I couldn't look her in the eyes. She was a bit shorter than me, even more so since I had three-inch wedges on. Her eyes were dark, only matched by her hair. When she smiled her face glowed and one small dimple graced her cheek.

Her name was Manny.

Within hours we had a date set for the very next day. My head was spinning. What was I doing? How would I face her? What if she tried to kiss me?

We picked a place that was right down the street from my work. A local hipster hangout that had pitchers of beer and a great vegan BLT. I took my time walking over, smoking enough cigarettes to make me look like a chimney. An amazing accomplishment considering it was a four-minute walk from my work.

I get to the café and see her standing outside next to her scooter. A little red thing with a black leather seat. She hugs me and says how great it is to see me. I smile, feeling my face turn red and my lungs turning black from all those damn cigarettes. I decide to take the "I'm too cool to say much" approach with her, when really my knees are knocking, my throat has closed up, my palms are sweating and my panties are only just beginning to get wet.

We find the place relatively empty and pick a seat up in the balcony. A table for four, she sits on the side with a cushiony bench, I sit across from her in a chair with my back to the café forcing me to have to keep direct eye contact.

I'm so nervous I can barely finish a sentence. I don't let her know this. I play it cool and quiet. She's charming, and I can see trouble written all over her face. We can smell our own kind. Her hands are small and delicate yet have a roughness about them. She's dressed in unlaced combat boots and jeans with a hoody. I can tell she has large breasts but hides them well. I start wondering what I could do to her body, and even better what she can do to mine.

After a couple of beers, she asks if I want to head back to her place. Why not? It's still daylight and I'm not accustomed to turning in early.

She hands me the second helmet to her scooter, and I just stand there staring. I give her a look, and she helps me put the helmet on. Getting close enough to me so I can smell her skin. My heart stops.

One terrifying scooter ride later and I'm standing in her living room getting the full tour of her apartment. She lives with a few roommates and I meet a couple of them. We get a few more beers and sit in her living room.

Her roommate sits with us chatting for a while, which I'm almost thankful for. I'm getting ever closer to facing my fear, and my body is all too aware.

He leaves.

She turns to me and forms a half smile, pulling the middle of her top lip into her mouth and wetting it with her tongue.

She puts her beer down on the coffee table, leaning in to kiss me. Her lips meet mine and I'm thankful I'm sitting down. Her lips are soft, with just the right amount of stickiness. She tastes like vanilla.

I hold my breath, unable to think of my next move. I feel like someone has grabbed onto my waist and pulled me hurtling backwards. I feel her hand on my face and know I haven't moved.

She pushes herself on top of me, never once parting her lips from mine. Her left leg moves to the outside of my right thigh, pushing her thigh against the crotch of my pants. My leg, I realize is doing the same to her.

Her hands have found their way onto my breast, her lips just hovering slightly over my ear. Soft moans coming from deep inside her.

We move into her bedroom. I find myself standing in front of her in just my panties, and she in panties and a sports bra. We resume the position we had been in on the couch, with less clothing to get in our way. I start understanding the logistics of it and don't feel as lost. Her bra falls off in the shuffle and I feel her warm large breasts against me. My panties get lost in the sheets, replaced quickly by her hand: soft and delicate yet firm and determined. I don't know if I had ever been this wet before. I want to giggle to myself at how effortlessly her fingers slide inside me.

She pulls back suddenly and says she'd really like to fuck me with a strap-on. I prop myself up on one elbow and look at her sheepishly. I still have to play coy, don't I?

I smile and say "What's keeping you, then?" She returns the smile and pulls out a purple strap-on. Fumbling for what feels like seconds, it's now attached to her in a black harness, condom on it, and she's ready to go.

I push her down on the bed and straddle her, the strap-on hitting the back of my ass. Leaning in to taste what vanilla still lingers on her lips, I grab hold of the strap-on and effortlessly slide it inside of me.

Her hands find their way up to my breasts, then down to my waist. In a low tone she tells me to fuck her like it's her dick. I start rocking my hips into her, picking up speed once I'm used to the hard feel inside of me.

Soon after, I witness my first female orgasm.

At that moment, I became an addict.

The next morning she gives me a ride to work on the same red scooter. Loaning me an ex-girlfriend's brown leather jacket, then deciding I should keep it. She pulls over outside my work and helps me off. She takes the helmet off of my head and kisses me. The vanilla is back and stronger than yesterday. I feel intoxicated from it.

I start to walk away. Turning around I catch the one-sided, dimpled smile. My own smile barely leaves my lips for the remainder of the day. My fear of women still lingers in my chest, but the throbbing between my thighs deafens it. Sometimes what scares us the most is what's hidden inside of us.

You Brought This on Yourself

Sandra D

I am an artist/craftsman/maker of beautiful things (just not babies). I am forty years old and I am still just a girl. I am a wife. I am an introvert. I am a rape survivor. I am infertile. I 'came of age' in the late '80s to early '90s, making my way from goth to grunge to granola in the process.

As a (virgin) teenager, I was a Good Girl. Honor Roll, part-time job, piano lessons and all. I had the usual crushes, stolen kisses and a couple of very respectful boyfriends, but I fantasized about being dominated. Like many Good Girls, I have always had thing for Bad Boys. In my younger days, I was persistently attracted to boys (and later, men) who frightened me, who were...a little rough. Any heavy petting I indulged in inevitably left me with bruises and I was proud of them, navel-gazing goth girl that I was. Those bruises proved there was blood in my veins, they made me feel edgy. They made me feel alive.

I was nineteen when I finally fell for a (married) man who was able to assuage just enough of my fear to convince me to give up my virginity. He maintained the upper hand by gently leading me down one kinky path after another, always keeping at the very edge of my comfort zone until he could tell me to do just about anything...and I would. He ended his marriage to be with me, though time would tell he could never actually be faithful to me. There were simply too many other women and men in the world to tempt his tastes. For all that, I somehow felt safe with him even though he made me uncomfortable. I got off on being just a little bit afraid. Like those early bruises, my discomfort made me feel edgy and alive, right up until I learned what 'against my will' really meant: the day I just didn't feel like having sex and he DID. Just because I lived with him and shared my bed with him did not mean I had forfeited my right to say no and it certainly did not give him the right to pin me to the floor and force me. That day was the beginning of the end for that relationship. I eventually realized that I spent most of my time in bed with him just waiting for it be over and the rest of the time dreading his touch, but it took me another year and a half to break away completely.

When I was twenty-one and before I had completed my breakaway, I went backpacking in Europe as do all good, middle-class college kids looking to broaden their horizons. After a night of too much drinking and bar hopping with people I didn't really know in a strange country, I fell prey again to that slightly frightened attraction. Unfortunately, this man was nothing like I had ever met before. When I said no, he simply beat me into unconsciousness and did what he wanted regardless. When I came to a few hours later, he was passed out. I grabbed my clothes, got back to my hotel to pack my bags and got myself out of town in a matter of hours. That was one set of bruises that brought me no pleasure or pride. Two towns later, I got myself to an English-speaking doctor who gave me a prescription for an antibiotic and a heaping serving of "You brought this on yourself, young lady" with nary a mention of counseling of any kind. Looking back, I do consider myself lucky. My attacker (I wonder, was he "mine"? Must I claim him? Surely I was not the only one to suffer at his hands?) only gave me herpes. He could have given me HIV/AIDS, he could have gotten me pregnant, he could have outright killed me. Lucky though I may have been, every time I have an outbreak, I relive that night in my head. And how very lucky, lucky, lucky that the Good Girl in me felt compelled to be upfront about the basics with every sexual partner that came after. Talk about a dampener.

Another year rolled by before I met the man who is now my husband. He was without a doubt a Bad Boy, from ponytail to police record and so on. Yet, here was another man that proved to be nothing like I had ever met before. This time, that meant that he was solely focused on my pleasure and my enjoyment. He never pushed me out of my comfort zone. Instead he made me feel not only safe, but cherished, and eighteen years later he still does. He IS my comfort zone. Sex in our marriage is not about who has the upper hand, pushing boundaries, asserting control or proving that I am alive. Sex is now a source of comfort in times of stress, it is soothing and relaxing. It is full of fun and often, laughter. It is intimate without any hint of violation and it is everything I need it to be.

BROKEN

Kate Anon

I am a thirty-one-year-old late bloomer. While I think I spent my teen years completely preoccupied by sex, it was not until I was almost nineteen that I finally acted on my desires. I can be found at @KateAnon and KateAnon.com.

In my early twenties, I struggled as a young woman married to a man with a very low libido. I was disappointed by married sex. I questioned if I was a sex addict, or had an unhealthy relationship with the act.

It was only after a few months of trying to conceive that I realized just how much of a problem *he* had. When you first decide to head down this road, you anticipate having intercourse all the time, to up your odds. When a man has his heart set on being a dad but doesn't want to do the act necessary to get things started, you worry. Hurdle one.

After visiting a urologist, we realized he made almost no testosterone. Which meant he produced almost no sperm. Hurdle two, which took years to properly discover. So, at twenty-five and thirty-nine, we became infertility patients. Shots and blood work for both of us. Restrictions on our sex life so we would be best able to move forward with

IVF.

We could no longer have sex for pleasure. It seemed all about creation. It wasn't pleasurable, anyway. Sex was now a reminder that we were broken. It reminded me of miscarriages and failed cycles and gained weight. It reminded him of low desire and lower hormone levels. It made us both feel like failures.

Our first IVF cycle, I hyperstimulated and wound up in the emergency room. Our next, the sample had no sperm; testosterone replacement is a delicate game and that round, we lost. We did finally go through cycles that seemed successful, until the time came to do the pregnancy tests. We were never able to conceive this way, because after starting a new regimen of drugs, an ultrasound showed an abnormal growth in my uterus. Hurdle three, and this one was the kicker: cancer.

My marriage was crumbling under the weight. We had been married for four years at this point, and before all this, I would have told you that we were a strong couple. I guess we just weren't strong enough.

I had always struggled with my sexual identity. I don't think I was very promiscuous, but my husband had only one partner before me, and I worried he did think that of me. I had always wanted more, kinkier, different. He preferred a regular schedule of missionary, not too often. I thought he'd come around, he just hadn't had enough experience to become experimental.

Boy, was I wrong. As we headed down the road of infertility treatments and disappointment, the sex happened less and less frequently. From about six months into trying to have a child, we were seeing doctors, so the only thing that would have resulted in a baby was insemination or IVF. With that fact in mind, my husband began to decline the invitation more and more.

Even my masturbatory habits became an issue. I'd have to hide it from him, and he'd shame me for wanting it. When we did try to have sex, things didn't work as they should, and he'd shut down from embarrassment. I would then resent him for not trying to please me, or not working harder to find a solution. No amount of Viagra can help when it's hormonal and psychological.

After almost two years of little to no sexual contact from my husband, I met a man. I did not want to be the clichéd adulteress, but I found myself quickly going down that road. No one had touched me, really touched me, in so long. I hadn't felt wanted in years. Here was someone who wanted me, who desired me, who wanted me to feel pleasure. I was not strong enough to resist, and with many justifications, I didn't want to.

As I started chemo, and wondered how much life I had left, I determined I wouldn't spend it frustrated and pining for what could have been. I carried on relationships for months with a couple of men. Men who were also in marriages like mine, which made me feel safer, made me feel better.

I don't make excuses for what I did. I know I was wrong. However, I won't continue to condemn myself for it. I truly believe it's one of the reasons I survived a time in my life that was pretty unbearable. As I finished cancer treatment and closed the door on having children, my husband knew I was unhappy and wanted a divorce. He attempted to initiate sex, the first time in more than three years, because he thought that would fix it. As if one act, after years of sexual neglect, could solve the problem. That's when I knew it was time to leave. That's when I knew that sex was important to me, important enough to make me stand up and say, "I deserve better."

I deserve love, passion and a good sex life. I think things may have been accelerated by our medical issues. Without them, it may have taken years for me to realize that we were completely incompatible sexually. I resolved to never make that mistake in a relationship again.

I'M A JANE

Jane Johnson

Jane is a stay at home mom. She used to teach middle school math a long time ago but has since forgotten the quadratic equation after hearing "Elmo's Song" one too many times.

Society dictates that no 'good' girl would want to fuck a John. When I found out that my boyfriend's sexual past included call girls, I wasn't shocked, I was curious. I've never seen prostitution or any other kind of sex work as an inherently bad thing in and of itself. In college and grad school, I was often regretful that a fat girl would never get work as an exotic dancer. Had I known then that there was a market for my body type, I would've been turning tricks in hotels instead of checking guests into them.

Maybe I'd seen *Best Little Whorehouse in Texas* a few

too many times, but I've always been troubled by narrative of the exploited prostitute as the definitive, or only, narrative. It is paternalistic to think that every woman involved in prostitution is a passive victim. It is patronizing to assume that no one would ever choose to be a prostitute, or that it could be a career that didn't involve exploitation.

I'm not completely naïve. I know that sex work has a lot of potential for abuse. In part, this can be caused by exploitation of the women involved. However, the police are also accountable in part-while both prostitution and solicitation are illegal, prostitutes are more frequently targeted in sting operations. Rape, theft and abuse go unreported. The public gleefully slut shames a sex worker. In articles about 'prostitution rings', the women are named, but not their patrons. A former sex worker could go on to win a Nobel Prize and every article about her would refer to her as a 'former prostitute.' For some, it is a career that will define – or end – their lives. For some, it will be a terrible experience. But not for all.

Once I knew I was in the bed of a John, I wanted to know about his experiences. I wanted to know if I was right that prostitution could be just another legitimate career choice. Perhaps I'd merely been brainwashed by one too many viewings/readings of a story involving the "hooker with a heart of gold" trope? From him, I learned about the world of independent call girls. Women who utilized their body as their business, controlled the pricing of their services, and chose which clients to see. Women who required a referral from another sex worker before they would see a client. Women who were not exploited. I couldn't be sure, though, how much of what he told me was narrative from the girls versus reality.

When I began writing a sex blog, I quickly plugged into that community. I developed friendships with a number of people working in the sex industry: phone sex workers, prostitutes (male and female), Johns, erotica authors, dancers and more. From any number of them, I began to piece together another narrative, one that straddled the middle ground, where sex workers could be independent and could do the work because they loved it, but one where they still occasionally took clients they didn't necessarily enjoy. I learned about what it was like to hide your work from your family (or not to), what sex worker activism looks like and why it is necessary. For many, it was like any other job, one that had its wonderful moments and its horrible moments, only without health insurance or predictable income.

Later that year I told my partner that I missed having sex with other women. I was very aroused by the idea of having sex with him and another woman. As it was also arousing to him, we began to discuss if it was a realistic fantasy to explore, and how best to do it.

The idea of hiring a professional was floated. Enjoyable sex without the stress and hassle of a relationship sounded appealing. Between my partner and my online community, I had the tools I needed to take the steps to find and hire a call girl.

I have patronized two women as a client, and hired a third on behalf of my husband while he was on a business trip. Much as I look for certain qualities in a pediatrician, I look for certain things in a call girl. I look for women who run their own websites. Who write copy that I find appealing. Who respond to emails professionally and within a reasonable amount of time.

It is a trope that men are visual and women want an emotional connection. It is also one that accurately describes me. When I am talking with a call girl, I don't want to waste her time (as it is as valuable as mine), but I do want to see if we can connect. Do I like her sense of humor? Do we share a common interest? No, I don't need (or deserve) to know her life story, her hopes and dreams, or the name on her driver's license. But I do want to have an experience that is enjoyable for all involved.

Plenty of Johns want to get right to the action, if their reviews of independent call girls are to be believed (and I do take them with a grain of salt). I tend to book an amount of time that allows for us to talk first. To warm up to one another before clothes are removed. For me, it's important to find a connection that makes me comfortable having a sexual experience with another person. Which is why I've never done well in a bar/club scenario: too loud to even be sure of someone's name, much less what book they last read.

Yes, part of the experience is awkward. It is strange to go to a hotel room, or a stranger's apartment knowing that you're going to have sex. It is awkward to hand over the money, which is why I'm glad it happens first. The first few moments (unless we are a repeat customer) are very much an awkward first date.

It has been my luck to meet intelligent, funny and sensual women who excel at dispelling that awkwardness. I've been lucky enough to patronize women who are happy to share and give tips on things like giving a spanking, or to instruct me in a new skill. These women have enriched my sex life, which is the exact opposite of what opponents of sex work would have me believe. I am a better lover and my marriage is stronger for these experiences.

While I am lucky to have had these experiences, I don't share them in such frank terms. I have technically broken the law. While I feel as though I can safely call for things like the decriminalization of prostitution, I do not feel as though I can openly call for them as a Jane. I think that if I came out as a Jane, my opinions on the topic would be dismissed, because (in part) I would no longer be calling for them as a (perceived) upstanding citizen/morally upright woman.

We don't seem to be capable of having an honest discussion about prostitution in the US. A veil of silence surrounds prostitution. Once the veil is lifted, the moralizing begins. We color interaction with a prostitute as a moral failing: that it somehow proves an immoral character. We paint prostitutes as everything from fallen women to victims, without ever painting them as feminists or as empowered. Society expected me to shame my partner for his past.

The narrative about prostitution is broken. Until we can admit the full spectrum of experiences as a prostitute, and as a John/Jane, we're not going to have an honest discussion about it, or be able to address any of the flaws or abuses. But if I'm being honest, I have too much lose to be the person to try to fix it publicly. I own that my silence is part of the problem, but that it is the right choice for me at this time.

HEALING THROUGH SAFE BDSM

Maple Muffins

I started having relationships in the early '90s. I gave my first blow job in 1992 and had sex for the first time in 1994. I work in environmental education, am married and am a mother.

I'm a kinky submissive. It's taken me a long time to be able to acknowledge that: both that I need that in sex, and what the definition of that is to me.

I came to BDSM in my early teens (in the '90s), by way of an abusive relationship. I didn't know at that time, what BDSM was, that it existed, or the difference between consent and abuse. What I did find, was amid the horror and controlling behavior, was that there were things I really enjoyed.

I was fourteen. This was my first sexual relationship, beyond groping and making out. The control had already begun before we even had sex the first time. He had narrowed down who I could speak to, what I could wear, etc.

He began to tell me however, what he'd read about control online (in those very early days of the internet). He was sixteen and in his youth definitely didn't know what was meant by safe, sane and consensual. What he did know was what he saw about control and humiliation excited him, and he was going to try it on me.

Little things started, like having me unbutton my shirt all the way while we drove around. He would knock down my appearance, point out my fat spots, and tell me what I could eat. I was dejected enough that I eventually did whatever he would say and even became anorexic.

Our first time having sex wasn't consensual; it also

wasn't very interesting, to be honest. He got more creative after that however. He'd have me go down on him while we drove (being teens we drove around a lot), forcing my face down so I couldn't breathe. We would find as public of places as possible like access roads to airports, beaches under a blanket, or back hallways in malls. I remember once his cupping and flaunting my breast for an older man who drove by us, then backtracked to see more. I began to feel a mix of shame and excitement in the exhibitionism. I still enjoy being shown off.

I was strictly not allowed to speak to other boys (upon threat of death. Yes, death), and he would often choke me during sex, telling me that I belonged to him, and that he would silence my whore mouth.

He would control my orgasms, and found great excitement in training me to cum on command. I still remember the mortification and the flush of heat in my face as he'd whisper, "cum now" in my ear at say...dinner with his parents. They must've thought me very odd!!

I eventually found the strength to leave him, as the death threats and physical attacks got worse. I found my way into a couple of boring vanilla relationships and realized...I really enjoyed being controlled.

I found myself sixteen and seeking another

controlling relationship (still not quite knowing a name for BDSM), and found myself again in another abusive one. This one extended itself into beatings, beyond the verbal abuse and rape. I found I loved a good spanking, but ultimately my sense of self-preservation won and I left for greener grasses.

Confiding in a friend about my conflicting feelings I was, at eighteen, introduced to a series of erotica novels which... Blew. My. Mind. I realized yes, THIS is what I want. I began to learn more about the 'right' way for things to work, how to play safely. I experimented. I had a gropefest with my two best friends. I slept with women. I ultimately loved men who could take an upper hand and still respect me.

Fast forward many years to today, I have really come into my own. I know what I want, and how to achieve it safely. I became a feminist who found sexual empowerment by giving over control in the bedroom...while still holding control of myself. I think some women unfamiliar with the lifestyle see BDSM as abuse, but having experienced it both ways, it is truly not the same thing at all! That information should be out there. It is not abuse if you are consensual, if you trust your partner, and safety mechanisms are set in place. It took me over a decade to realize that difference. I can enjoy now, a good spanking, control, a little humiliation, and know that it can all stop at my word. I've been asked if I would make different choices if I could go back, and I wouldn't! Those experiences made me who I am, and I still find some of the thoughts tantalizing. There is healing in safe BDSM.

FUCKED UP AND GLORIOUS

Hopper James

I am finally single at thirty-seven years old, twice divorced. I work in IT project management, but I moonlight as a fiction editor. I love writing, but career-wise my aspirations are in editing. Also, I'm kinky as hell and don't plan on settling down again.

I packed twelve different panties for three days at a Leather conference.

The cutest and laciest pair I brought got ripped by something involving chains whilst in my suitcase, so they were totally out of the question for the Friday night play party and I didn't like the rest of them as much, so I went entirely without. I thought nothing of this as I donned a shimmery black miniskirt, slit to my hip; garters and fishnets, and an oddly comfortable PVC corset, which I had lubed until it was glassy. In patent leather knee-high boots, I didn't cut too poor a figure. My shoulders were square, my posture straight. I could probably pull off a bit of a strut: you know, throw a swing in my step. Something in between "boots made for walkin'" and "for a good time, call..."

Swagger and all, I was beyond butterflies-excited for this party. We had met a few months before this convention, and she and I had engaged since in an echo of flirtation, exchanging messages slippery with innuendo. We understood each other, had excellent synchrony. Not hurting the process were those friends who nudged and encouraged. A mutual friend handed me a cup of coffee and named her "The Sadist's Sadist." This designation made my belly drop into my cunt with hope and heat and maybe some fear. I was well aware that my reputation for algolagnia preceded me. The competition for the mantle of "pain slut" especially one able to orgasm from the pain, was one where I was the only entrant. It's sheer hedonism, fucked up and glorious. The downside to this kink were the times I stopped myself from saying to a lackluster top, "Yeah, thanks for playing with me! No, I didn't come, you couldn't hurt me well enough."

But *she* played hard. I played hard. And we were a promising match on complementary ends of the whip, or flogger, or whatever the hell she wanted to wield.

From a balcony in the hotel's atrium, I spied her as she mingled below. Her amazing curve emphasized by a black leather cincher, she looked delicious. I had fuck all idea how much feasting would ensue.

I mentioned to her what I had heard: her expertise, she's a natural, the appreciation people in the scene have for the way she fucks up girls. The word '*beaming*' nearly does justice to her reaction.

We met up an hour or so later, she had doffed her pointy blue suede shoes, her bare feet were pedicured and pretty. She stood at the top of a flight of stairs and stared down at me, grinning. As I approached, she declared her hunger. She led me towards the women's play space, which was a new thing to me. I love women and played only with women, but always in trans spaces. I sensed a difference. She warned me that the feel of the room wasn't totally up to speed, it was early, but we'd change that. I followed her as she dragged a chair around: the right vibe was essential. When she found the place she liked the best, she directed someone to move a bench out of the way, pointing. The girl complied post-haste. We stood facing and she pulled me into her arms. We centered, together. We briefly spoke in safety terms, reviewed what was agreed-upon. She asked me about how it was to orgasm from pain.

"Is it, like, to release pain, to get past it, through it?"

I replied plainly: "Not like that, no. Pain is what makes me come."

She just nodded, and didn't let on that I had scored a point. I didn't realize that she had a desired answer until much later, when we were whispering following the violence and basking in the afterglow.

She takes my hands, flexes my wrists. Quickly, she turns me to face away and twists my arm up behind me, and then bends my wrist somewhichway enough to make me gasp.

It's on. We're doing this.

She unlaces my corset a bit, pausing to bite my shoulder blade so hard that her teeth were still on my back the next night. She pinched the inside of my left arm, where I have tattooed wings, assuring me it will mark. With the bites and pinches, I edge towards climax, and fuck fuck fuck, it hurts. Pinching is never easy for me to process. I'm unused to it. I try to tell myself it's not because it's out of my league, it's just out of my ken. This isn't canes, this isn't tools. This is hands. *Her* hands.

She motions. I take the chair, she kneels.

The juxtaposition is not lost on me.

Her first strikes to my inner thighs are no cuddly preamble, no BDSM 101 warm-up. In near-panic I push her hands away. Wait, just..!

"Hold on to the chair."

Ok. A job, a task; I can do that. I can. She hits my thighs again.

And then she stops.

"You're not wearing underwear."

I want to explain the reason. She gives me no time to speak.

"*Girls* wear underwear. Dirty. Little. Sluts. Don't." She slaps my thighs, right, left, right, right, punctuating each word. "Are you a dirty little slut?" She purrs, wanting my confession.

"Maybe?" I squeak.

"Maybe?" thudstingslap. "*Maybe?*" Again.

"Yes?" I try again, giggling.

"Yes. Yes. You are." I gasp with the pepper of blows.

I come with no warning, shivering.

Admittedly, there was some point in the progress of this scene where she directed I should only orgasm with permission. Admittedly, I can't remember where in the storm that was. Admittedly, I didn't ask every time. When I remember to ask again she doesn't say yes.

"Not yet." Her rhythm doesn't stutter, she doesn't even look up to deny me.

This is more than a little aggravating. I clench my jaw, trying to hold back the impending wave.

She has a tiny paddle that fits in her hand. It's plastic or plexi or something. Whatever it is, it's *bitchy*. She works my thighs for some time with it; it's breathtaking. I am not sure how to get through it. When she offers me the choice between her continuing with the tiny paddle or her hands (open and clenched), I want her hands. Not because this is any easier to process, it's probably not, but I want the connection. I want her touch, however sinister the delivery. When my eyes are open, I am looking at the hollow of her throat, her mouth, her eyes. I don't look at her hands, but I know they move fast.

She says, as she slaps my chest, punches my chest, that she was going to hurt my thighs more, but I'm taunting her.

"It's like your chest is calling to me," She says, punching my thigh, then my chest. One-two. Left-right.

I am overwhelmed. The expanding wave of orgasm was fast becoming a tsunami. Some of this is decidedly catharsis, but overwhelmingly a wall of feelings from not only pain, but her continual mockery of me.

This is her delight, she's *enjoying* me.

I feel so good and pretty.

It's big. I gasp.

"I need a moment." I use words.

I want to collect the tsunami and tuck it behind my ear, deal with it later. She checks in with me, holds my face, makes sure I see her, see her. She says, "we're here, it's good. It is good. It's so good."

"But. Just. Can I have a minute?" I say again, somewhat woozy.

"That's why we're talking, you know. You're getting a minute." She smiles. She makes sense, but my own sense-making is slipping away like the tide right before that really big wave.

She continues her assault, having granted me the chance to catch my breath. My legs are marked, they are red and purple and black, the bite on my back bites back every time I lean into the chair.

I don't usually mark. It takes a certain something, and I don't know the equation.

I am making noises, I know, and some is an unrelenting orgasm, some is how loud I ache. After a little longer, I'm unsure of holding back the wave that I have behind my ear and my breath hitches. The flood of tears is loosed and she stops and puts her arms around me, and I cry and babble into her hair and neck and hope I don't get mascara all over her white shirt. She speaks soothing things, in soothing tones.

With our foreheads steepled, she says:

"You're giving me your tears. What an amazing gift. And look, here are mine." She is moved, this is for her, too. I blissfully smile, I am tired and wish I could be in her grip of pain for longer, for longer. I am past a cliff, near wordlessness. She gathers me up a bit, dispatching someone to bring me water. I sit, breathing, blinking. Smiling, sniffling.

We are exhausted and exhilarated. I wrap up in a blanket and drink, she gives me chocolate.

She has a special present, she does, in that I do not cry for anyone else, and never have from pain. She has a special presence, she does, in that I can't deliver expression from nowhere, this was skillfully elicited, compelled, drawn from me. Her force in the destruction of my levees and dams and locks, the will she exerted in granting my ecstatic agony, driving me to a perfectly exquisite, blinding pain.

The kind that makes everything afterwards much easier to see.

DIRTY LITTLE SEX

Foxy Kitten

Happily married mid-western housewife.

I'm a total control freak. I can't handle things not being "just so." That is how I cope with stress. I hide in controlling all aspects of my life and my household.

But in the bedroom? I'm a complete submissive.

A lot of people don't understand the psychology

behind the desire to submit. For the longest time I didn't understand it either. I thought I was a freak or that something was wrong with me. I now know that I'm fine. Think about it: what would be the ultimate pleasure and relaxation for someone who feels the compulsive need to control every aspect of life? Giving up that power. Sex is purely about pleasure. So naturally, the most enticing thing in the world to the control freak in me is to have all of my control taken away, in a safe and consensual environment, of course!

My first experience with BDSM was in my twenties with a 'friend with benefits.' He was commanding, confident and just fucking sexy. When I told him that I was into submission you would've thought I had just let loose a kid in a candy store. He was a natural dominant.

When I think of our encounters certain things stick out in my memory...

- Laying on the golf course of our country club at night, with two of his fingers shoved deep into my throbbing pussy. Him whispering through gritted teeth into my ear, "This belongs to me! I am going to tease you for hours and only let you cum when I'm good and fucking ready."

- A sixty-nine in the back seat of my car. I could barely get his cock in my mouth. He was *huge*. Like, porn star huge. And he knew how to work his tongue. He did this thing where he would stick his tongue deep inside me and use his nose to bump my clitoris.

- Him bending me over the hood of my car and smacking my ass, then turning me around and shoving three fingers into my wet pussy. I gasped and told him three was too much. He responded, "No it isn't. You can take it. This isn't about your pleasure, it's about mine and you'll do as I tell you. Don't ever tell me 'no' again." I had never been so turned on before.

The very first time we had intercourse. It was the night after I was date raped. I went to him and told him about it because I knew that he was a man that I could trust. He turned my chin up to him, looked me in the eyes and said, "I will never make you do anything that you don't want to." I cried and kissed him. Then I gave him head. He chastised me for not yet knowing how to deep throat, a skill I would master later. I got on top to ride him and I experienced something I've never experienced since. He was so big that the feeling it gave me was a weird mixture of pain and pleasure. It was amazing.

We had some great, sexy times, but we were terrible as a couple.

The only man who has ever turned me on more is

my wonderful husband! He's the only man to find my g-spot and the only man to ever give me an orgasm. There was just a crazy, primal attraction between us. It really is like our bodies were made for each other.

We communicate really well and that's the most important part of making any type of relationship work.

My husband isn't as into BDSM as I am, but I have slowly introduced the blindfolds, restraints and paddles, and he has agreed to use them, much to my pleasure! He has said that he never wants to speak degradingly to me or really hurt me. I've got to respect that. I don't want to be called a slut anyway. I prefer dirty little sex kitten.

THAT MIRANDA

Elis Bradshaw

I am a writer by calling and an administrative assistant by profession; I was also a semi-professional bike racer for a handful of years, but that didn't pay the bills. I was born in 1981, and I really started exploring my sexuality

*in the late nineties, in a rather conservative small town.
The conservative part meant that there were tremendous
expectations of premarital chastity and heterosexuality
and the small-town part meant that there was a lot of sex
happening, much of it casual.*

It wasn't a great idea, and I knew it. Miranda was
straight; even if she hadn't been, she didn't like me
much. Still, when she pointed at me and
announced to our friends that I'd be sleeping with
her that night, I didn't protest. I followed her up the
stairs to her room, I slipped into her bed.

Bad idea or not, I wanted it. I'd known I was
bisexual for years by the time I found myself in
Miranda's bed, and I had made good headway into
the world of boys. Boys were easy. Girls, though,
were tricky. I'd taken part in my female friends'
sexual experiments but it had never gone beyond
kissing and copping a feel over their shirts. They
usually brushed my hand away; that's how it is
when you're trying to get some from straight girls.

By the time Miranda announced that she was
taking me into her bed that night, I was long
overdue for some girl action. I'd only drunk once
before, and whatever had been in the red cup
someone handed me trickled straight down
between my legs. Heat and liquor spread through

my crotch, and while a few clumsy spin-the-bottle kisses took the edge off, I couldn't wait to get upstairs and into her bed. And her pants.

I hadn't given much thought to Miranda before that night, but once I had my hands on her I realized just how much I loved her body. Lean and lithe with an androgynous streak, her figure posed a stark contrast to my rounded lines. Compact breasts at the top of her chest, skin tight over her hipbones. I covered one of her breasts with my palm while I kissed her, then leaned down and took her nipple into my mouth. Her skin rippled with goosebumps as I drew tiny circles with the tip of my tongue.

Tentatively, I moved my hand down and nudged my fingers under her waistband. I paused to gauge her reaction. So far so good; I pressed further, grazing her pubic hair. The Brazilian hadn't yet come into vogue, and her bush was full and thick. Luxurious. She tensed as my fingers passed over her clit, then relaxed as I gave a few light strokes. I opened her up and pushed one finger inside of her. She was so, so warm inside. Soft and thick and sticky.

I took her pants off and put them at the foot of her bed. My first licks were small and shy. I'd like to say I was teasing her and building tension, but the reality is that never having gone down on a woman before, I just didn't know what I was doing. I needed to start out slow. I was surprised at how different our pussies looked. Miranda had short labia that fanned out far in the middle, making a pink half-moon, mine were thick all the way along their length and dusty purple.

As desire overpowered my inexperience, I grew bolder and more animated. I traced her whole pussy with my tongue, testing different textures. Wet skin, slick hair, the hard little bump of her clit. I pushed my tongue inside of her and tasted meat and salt. Miranda coated my tongue.

She moved underneath me and I wanted so badly to make her come. I used my fingers, my mouth; when I came up for air I kissed her so she could taste herself. I returned to her breasts, breathing on them so her nipples stood up and her gooseflesh came back. I loved watching her body respond to me.

The drinks I'd had and the newness of the positions – so different from being with a boy – combined and made my head spin. Kissing my way back up her body, I laid back on my pillow for a moment, one hand still stroking her breasts. Miranda reached between my legs and began to stroke me. Lightly, gently, then a little quicker. It didn't take long, just a minute or two; I came. Hard, clenching her hand between my legs, rocking my hips back and forth with every last little shudder. The last thing I remember is wanting to make her feel what I'd just felt, to make her come and cry out. Then, just like a boy losing his virginity, I fell asleep.

When I woke up, it was later than I expected. I was tucked into a ball on the far side of her bed and Miranda was gone.

SCHEHERAZADE

Kate Conway

During the day, I edit freelance work and provide customer support for a start-up in the San Francisco Bay Area. I'm also the Queer Studies Editor at xoJane.com. In my spare time, I frequently write fiction and poetry, take improv and voice-acting classes, fail at running half-marathons, and explore all the nooks and crannies of the great city of San Francisco.

I'm twenty-two, so I guess you could say I came of age basically yesterday. This story takes place when I was in high school in the mid-2000s.

You can find me on Twitter at @KatChatters.

Maybe all high school romances are like this, all searing heat and bitten nails, and me and Audrey were no exception. Audrey never knew how to love a little bit, only in intense, sharp bursts. We spent most of late August in parking lots, sitting in her 1989 Camry, slipping around on the cracked leather seats as sweat slicked the backs of our thighs.

"Tell me a story," she'd say, seat leaned back as far as it would go and feet kicked up on the dash. I'd watch as her uniform skirt puddled around her thighs, tan and strong from lacrosse. She'd follow my gaze down to her lap and smile, stretch, rub her ankles together where her feet pressed up against the windshield. I'd swallow.

Audrey and I liked to play a game where we refused each other everything, and I'd play it then, leaning back against the passenger-side door and sliding my sunglasses down my nose. "You tell me one."

She'd wrap a hank of my then-long hair around one callused palm and tug, not hard, just enough to sting. "I'm bored, Kate," she'd remind me as I melted toward her, open-mouthed. "You're the only one who isn't boring."

I'd smile against her then, swiping my tongue over the salty skin behind her ear, daring, wanting, afraid. "So give me something to talk about."

The whole time, she'd keep my hair wound around her wrist like a talisman.

While cleaning out my room in my parents' house, I find a stack of letters, creased and soft. I read them quickly, barely taking any of them in, save a passage here and there.

I loved you so much, I think, but things got intense so fast. I keep having nightmares where the stories I write are real, that I wake up and I'm forty and married and unhappy and dull. I think you'd be happy like that, which is worse. Please don't be mad at me, but I think you'd be happy like that.

Audrey wrote like a Dorothy Parker character without any of the self-awareness. But at the time these had gutted me, left me staring and trembling in the senior bathroom, and they gut me now.

They weren't all breakup letters. We each used to leave notes in the other's locker, tucked among binders and empty coffee cups. I'd grab for my science binder and watch a crumpled ball of notebook paper tumble out. It'd open into a doodle of Audrey asleep on a desk, captioned "I HATE EVERYONE EXCEPT YOU AND HOLDEN CAULFIELD." They make a pile in my lap, some funny, some cranky, all of them only ours.

"I'll take you home today," says one of the notes in thick, rounded magenta Sharpie. I remember this one.

She'd hand-delivered it to me in fifth period, bold as you please, hair spilling out from her ponytail over the shoulders of her stiff uniform shirt. "Message from the office for Kate?" she chirped, sliding it across my desk before our English teacher could get it away from her.

Not that Ms. Falway would have even thought to: I was a compulsively good student, a people-pleaser, biting my lip with nerves before every test and leaving sweaty palm-prints on every page of *Catcher in the Rye*. I tried to keep my expression neutral even so, though, dragging my eyes away from the backs of Audrey's knees as she left.

"Good news from the office?" Ms. Falway chirped

above me, and I stuffed the note down into my bag and grinned, trembling.

"Just...soccer practice got canceled." A stupid lie, easily cross-checked, but who cared. Only Audrey, and she hadn't stuck around to know the difference.

After school, I lingered at my locker, sliding the palms of my hands along the cool metal walls until the last of the chatter had faded from the halls. Audrey was perched on the hood of her car when I got there, her aviators on. She looked like the star of an '80s movie, all battered notebook and charm, and I told her so.

She laughed. "God, you're cliché."

I stopped, swallowed. "Sorry."

"Oh, I'm just kidding," she dismissed. "I'm glad you came."

"I'm skipping Student Council for this," I said stupidly, and her eyes went dark and intent.

"Good," she said. She slid off the hood and swung the driver's-side door open, motioning for me to get in the passenger seat. She watched, waiting, as I struggled with the seatbelt. In the car, the silence was thick.

"So," she said when I finally got myself situated. "Where do you want to go?"

"Oh, well, home," I said. "Or...My mom's not expecting me for an hour at least."

"Yeah," she said, pulling out of the parking lot and heading for nowhere in particular.

I loved when Audrey kissed me, her thin lips always sun-chapped and salty, and this time was no exception. She fisted my collar as soon as we parked, yanking me toward her and making me scrabble at the seatbelt, choking.

"Jesus, Audrey," I said, and she bit my lip. I went quiet.

It was still so hot in Sacramento, and my shirt clung to my back as Audrey yanked it from the waistband of my skirt, sliding her hands up to palm at my bra with something like wonder.

"My boobs are small," I said apologetically, and she shook her head. Moved by some daring, I cupped both of hers before ducking my head under the hem of her shirt to bite at one nipple. It tasted just like the rest of her – sweaty, sun-screened – but it made me breathless all the same. She gasped above me, and I grinned as she knotted her fingers in my hair.

"Should we...backseat?" I asked, peeking at her face, which was high-cheekboned and flushed. She nodded, then shook her head.

"No, let's...can we..." She moved sideways to brace

against the driver's-side door, and I moved between her legs, kissing her bottom lip again before edging my hand under her skirt.

"Can I?" I said, and she nodded, looking away. I didn't kiss her again, only watched her face as I slid my hand up her knee, farther, where her thighs got soft and where she was friendly and damp.

"Yes, please, Kate," she said, urgent. I pressed my hand against the wetness in her underwear, the way I liked to do to myself in my bedroom, thinking of this, thinking of the way her breasts pressed against her shirt in geometry class, the way she'd trail one hand over my shoulder as she passed me on the way to lunch.

She used to leave me hickeys there along my collarbone for me to examine later, laying the pad of one finger over the purple spot for good luck, feeling it pulse as I crossed and uncrossed my legs in English class, aching.

That same intense pressure bloomed in my lower back as I touched Audrey, making me squirm even as she did the same.

She grabbed my wrist, digging her nails into the soft part of my forearm until I clumsily slipped my fingers underneath her cotton underwear, straight into the heat of her. I stopped for a minute, struck by the smell of her, copper and sour. It smelled like the way her mouth tasted when we kissed, all spit and teeth.

"What are you doing?" she gritted, and I crooked my two fingers, hesitant. It was so different to do this to someone else, to feel her clench and twitch around me, my thumb swiping against her clit as her thighs tightened on my hand, almost painful. The ridges inside her reminded me of tiny sea anemones, living quiet in the dark, and I scrabbled over at them, over and over, until my hand got sore.

"Like that," she said. It sounded almost hollow, like she knew what people said when they were close to coming. "Just like that."

I pressed deeper into her, the whole heel of my palm against her pubic bone, and she shuddered suddenly, opening. Her pussy, which had been tight and hard and pulsing, gave then under my hand, dripping like an overripe peach. I gulped, panting, and she moaned a little. Every sound she made twanged at me; every time I twisted my fingers, I imagined her doing the same to me, imagined my face between her legs, imagined her taking, taking, always taking.

"Do you want me to..." I started. I desperately wanted to know how she tasted, suddenly, but I couldn't imagine how to even start. I wanted her to hold me there, my hair held fast around her wrist. I wanted to choke on her.

I snuck another look at her face, but she wasn't looking at me. She was turned toward the window, eyes closed. As I watched, she breathed in through her mouth and arched, keening, grabbing hold of my hand again and forcing it against her. I waited for her face to crumple like paper left in the rain.

Afterwards, we drove to my house without speaking. Audrey put a Placebo song on repeat: Protégé Moi, Protégé Moi, Protégé Moi, and rolled the windows down. I looked out at the asphalt. Protégé moi.

"See you tomorrow!" I called to her as I shut the passenger-side door outside my front yard. She shook herself a little, as if coming out of a dream, and then smiled at me.

"See ya," she said, sliding her sunglasses down over her eyes and driving down the heat-shimmering street.

Wiping my hand on my skirt, I watched her leave.

THE SENSUALIST

Luisa Colt

The sensualist knows nothing without feeling. I have sought answers: a label, a framework to understand my sexuality, with the insecurity of an abandoned child. Without a cohesive identity to present to you I fear I have failed. Reliant on the most simplistic of structures – a chronological narrative – I will try to explain how it is I became this collection of paradoxes: a wife, a slave, a feminist, a white-collar professional, a stripper, a bisexual, and even sometimes, a prude.

The story starts as a young girl. Third year of elementary school, masturbating to orgasm under my school desk. Back row, squeezing my thighs together systematically to release. Flushed cheeks, ragged breathing, but finally, release. Looking around, nobody seemed to notice. Lunchtime, I knew different.

My mother brought 'educational' books home from the library and handed them to me silently. By then I was a competent reader and consumed them enthusiastically, alone. *Where Did I Come From?* depicted the practical act of lovemaking between a decidedly rounded husband and wife, but it raised more questions than it answered. If that rubenesque pair could kiss and cuddle and make all those love hearts appear – and a baby – and that's what sex was, what was it that I was doing? Sex education: anatomically correct cross-sections, abstractions of something that was consuming me whole. My tension wasn't just lying there, matter of fact on a page. I knew I wasn't making a baby. I was alone. None of it made sense.

Alone in my bedroom, under the cover of night and my Strawberry Shortcake doona, I loved to touch myself. As masturbation tends to go, it was a solitary pleasure that conjured a longing for company. I craved someone to acknowledge it. The closest I came was a sleepover. My best friend from pre-school and her other friends lay out mattresses on her living room floor. She mounted her pillow and playfully kissed and rode on it in front of all of us. We all had a turn. We created orgiastic dioramas with our (all female) Barbie dolls. When I think about it now I see those plastic limbs bent back, perfectly smooth junctures of legs and torsos bumped against each other to all of our delight.

Even now I feel the need to be very clear about something. I was never sexually abused. But like other young girls, I had intense feelings I navigated alone. I knew from the fact that nobody talked about it that it was something I should keep private. Silence corrupted the natural, stirred it into shame. I assumed, as children do, that there was something wrong with me. I felt that somehow I had instigated those childhood experiments with my dirty mind, that I had poisoned others by simply being there. It wasn't until the internet that I was relieved of this solitary burden.

Dial-up internet coincided beautifully with adolescence. Just turned twelve, a new girlfriend who wanted to share babysitting duties. The awkward grey Apple Macintosh woken while her younger siblings slept. We logged onto an adult chat room that she had found somehow. Outrageous statements of lust interspersed with smooth, angry looking hard-ons and pneumatic breasts. As soon as I got home I begged my mother to buy a modem. Homework of another kind: from the intellectual to the profane. Trawling the emerging web of raw erotic fiction, the delicious pain of downloading images bit by byte, a voyeur of volatile IRC chat rooms. All in the name of alchemy, creating and deciphering the intricate chemistry of sex.

Thirteen. My desire blossomed under blue light. The laughable pretext of police and adult supervision at the local scout hall: an alibi. The darkness: our collaborator. Pressed into a corner, ah, finally! Lips in tentative negotiation, tasting a home cooked dinner, ill-gotten booze on shallow breath, insistent fingers searching over, under clothes. Their hard cocks through their pants. Hard, slick with pre-cum. God, I was hungry. Hungrier than I felt those awkward boys were. Predatory. I craved a man in this proliferation of boys.

Blossoming confidence led me to a connection. The closest I had to a boyfriend for several years. Him: twenty-six, across the Atlantic, my sexual collaborator and confidante. Me: fourteen. Endless nights on IRC bookended with volumes of emails. Together, alone, touching ourselves to incremental conversations, frantic redials, urging each other to orgasm. Digital photography didn't exist, but a visual reference wasn't necessary. It was desire dealt in words. Finally: reality. His (surprise!) girlfriend found and seduced me artfully. She'd logged in as him, made me hungry and wet before unleashing a tirade of abuse. He found me on Facebook fifteen years later, but that's another story.

The same year I met a forty-nine-year-old online who lived in the same city. Emails for months before he asked me if I'd like to meet up. Even then, instinct served me well. I never saw that salt and pepper hair. Hysterics can point fingers at predators but to me the most important conversation about power is still not happening. Talk to girls about sex and pleasure. Fuck virginity, masturbation is the holy grail. The prize within your self: your pleasure, yours. It renders virginity irrelevant until loving commitment brings up the question. Empowerment. Total control. Self-worship. Had I been told masturbation was a precious gift I could – and should – give myself, I doubt I would have shared it and made myself vulnerable in this situation and others. I was incredibly lucky.

Overlay a blur of the usual high-school hysteria over boys, men in posters, guys in bands. Outwardly the all-girls' schoolgirl. Boys my age still mostly uninterested in anything outside of sports or academia. Imaginary courtships started in stunted one-word exchanges on the back seat of the bus. IRL sex with these boys was out of the question. Still, more anonymous exchanges at underaged parties, or house parties held by friends presented opportunities.

Careful to disguise myself, I never dressed provocatively. Dressed in loose jeans, oversized polo shirts and sneakers. Hair always tied back neatly in a pony-tail or bun. On recollection it was unfair to those poor boys. I would find a way to get them alone. Kiss them passionately. Slide my hand into their jeans. I always loved cocks, all shapes and sizes. Loved making them hard and wet with pre cum. Surreptitious grinding and exploratory manual adventures. Once I was done I craved none of the things my friends obsessed over. No desire for a boyfriend. I considered myself a sexual adventurer.

Fifteen: sex with my best friend. Her mother had now moved to an outrageously designed seventies mansion on the outer suburbs of our city. Again recruited to babysit her younger siblings. After sharing a bottle of awful, sweet Sangria on the heated carpet floor, we found her mother's bed, a stash of video-taped porn. The tangle of hormones and visual inspiration and sheer opportunity. The nervous electricity of first touches. Slowly undressing. Kissing impossibly soft lips. Smooth, bare skin and suckling breasts. Writhing in a sixty-nine, a hot, probing mess of tongues and fingers. I still remember her manicured long nails sliding inside me, hands I had always been envious of. I was in heaven...and woke in hell. Conspicuously alone. She was back in her bunk bed and wouldn't wake up to talk to me. With a raging hangover I walked to the train station and vomited in a trash can. I was crushed. I sat on the train in tears. Turning the house upside down in my mind for clues: am I gay? What have I done? Is she going to tell everyone? She apparently never did. We are still friends, but to this day she has never wanted to talk about it. The lasting impression fit perfectly into my suspicion that I had somehow engineered yet another situation to be ashamed of.

I waited eagerly again for weekends. Exploited the darkness. Waiting for an opportunity to arise with somebody who would go further. Not just anybody. A character that would inflame my imagination, stimulate my desire, who was strong enough to take me.

Finally: Sixteen. I decided my virginity had to go. It all started on a school ski-trip. The math teacher – who was also a tennis coach – had brought several fellow tennis coaches to chaperone. One of them was a college student a decade older than me who was reasonably cute, bookish, strong, interested but reluctant. After some very heavy making out sessions behind the jacuzzi room (snow, steam) I couldn't persuade him to take my virginity at camp. He promised to fuck me when we got back, if I was still interested. His place wasn't the college hangout you'd have expected: it was his parents' place. He had a waterbed. And I got exactly what I went there for.

Losing my virginity was pleasurable and, for me, a relief. I didn't lose it so much as strategically dispense of it. Moments of physical obsession, connection, and devastation don't need to be about love for me, though the many times I have had sex whilst in love are different again, another facet of the same brilliant phenomenon.

The idea that somehow I still was a virgin, despite everything I had thought, felt, and done seemed like a joke. So, the setting was unsentimental. The soundtrack was laughable. The waterbed, whilst a challenge, proved impossible. I wasn't fooling around. We moved to the floor, and finally, it was happening. Me on top. Stacks of books and whispered moans. He was shocked at how much I enjoyed myself. His words: "It can't feel that good." It did. It wasn't his skill. I smiled the whole way home. Again, I found myself on the train, the world speeding past me, transformed as if in a giant centrifuge, thinking how differently the world looked now. I couldn't believe there was a world out there comprised of people that did this all the time. Why did they spend so much time and effort covering it up? Pretending this wasn't the greatest thing ever?

Why do we?

We fucked in his shitty car, the cliffs on the beach near my house, the suburban park near his, then it was over. I wasn't interested in him as a boyfriend, no more than he was interested in having an underaged girlfriend. The next time I saw him was eight years later, when he'd started dating my then boyfriend's sister.

Her: "This is X."

Him: "Hey, don't I know you from somewhere?"

Me: "Yeah, you helped me lose my virginity!"

My boyfriend: "..."

Far from opening the door to promiscuity I merely settled back into regular school life. You can skim read this part, as there's no sex for two years. I still made out with those I found interesting at parties but there were no boyfriends and no sex. I silently judged my peers inadequate for anything but classroom or bus-stop cohabitation. In my final year of school I met a guy my own age online. He was creative, sensitive, sexually demanding. He lived on the other side of the world. His plan was to move to my country on a one-year working visa so we arranged to meet.

What began as a passionate, obstinate love affair became tempered with habitual negligence as the years passed. A year in my country, a year in his. I went to college, we got jobs. The sensitivity that had fascinated me in the early days of our relationship now seemed like weakness. I cooled towards him intellectually, became repulsed by the thought of sex with him.

Once he had received his permanent residency I left him and began to take on lovers. Without wanting a relationship I always saw something in them, or perhaps in me, that demanded the relentless exploration of connected mind and body for hours at a time.

On completing my degree I found an internship at a prestigious agency. They offered me a job almost immediately. Outwardly I was an accomplished graduate with a steady income and a bright future, but the image I presented was incompatible with my fundamental nature: fickle, curious, tempestuous. I was bored, suffocated, and half-living. In desperation I decided to move.

Moving to a new city was a shift of tectonic proportions. It birthed a continent within, one of dramatic mountain ranges and vast tracts of unexplored land. I had a new boyfriend, a place of my own, but I was finding it hard to find another job.

Then, the most vivid dream: a stage, bright lights, throbbing music, the deliberate uncoiling of a bra, oozing confidence, a wry smile.

Striptease.

On waking, I tentatively shared my dream with my then-new boyfriend. He'd known girls who were strippers before, in fact it was a big business in this city, and he thought I could do it. I had nowhere near the self-confidence I thought I'd need. I was still hiding myself under – slightly tighter – jeans and t-shirts. Yet there was something about the potential to become that goddess in my dream, and better yet to make the money I needed to survive.

Nerve-wracking doesn't even start to cover standing, almost knock-kneed on a red-lit stage, wearing six-inch heels for the first time, praying for twenty agonizing minutes to be over before you fall off. But taking your new, tiny clothes off isn't the scary part. Navigating the men and keeping your cool while dealing with constant (sometimes cruel) rejection was the harder skill to acquire.

The elaborate and necessary cultivation of a sexual alter-ego: first, you 'pick' a name ("No, not that one, it's taken. Not that one either. How about we just give you one, love?") Then hone a personality: mine was a peculiarly attractive combination of seductress/confidante/tease/bitch that mirrored my own. The club I worked at had a strict no-touching rule and drugs weren't tolerated. I was sexually potent, peppered with an intellectual curiosity, but ultimately safe. I interacted with all types of men, discovering one by one the different triggers and tastes they wore so close to their wallets.

After several months I'd had an education money couldn't buy. I could read a room in sixty seconds, find a target, and take what I wanted. The money was more than I could ever – or can still – make in my tertiary educated desk job. A litmus test for societal hypocrisy. Grueling hours buoyed by a huge roll of tax-free cash. Independent financially, and professionally considered a contractor, nobody told me how hard to work, when to work, who to dance for. Feline, predatory, untouchable. Not taking shit from anyone, even if they'd paid me. Even, no, *especially* if they'd emptied their bank account. At the slightest offence, I walked.

Those four years were like a second adolescence. The foundation built inside the club led to my redefining emotional and sexual boundaries. Self-respect. Self-protection. Loving and caring for myself. I don't pretend it wasn't a risky proposition. Then, I always did like the deep end.

I think you are either tough going into the sex industry, or you get tough, and tough isn't a bad thing. Necessity is a powerful motivator. Dispensed of body hang-ups: there is always going to be an appreciator of your particular configuration of parts. Learning to wield the power I had over men...and women. Beyond necessity, the flourishes of intricate, lasting beauty of mind. Owning my confidence unapologetically. Building and holding boundaries in (real or imagined) intimacy. Appreciating rather than being intimidated by other women's success. Things I rarely see replicated outside the club's four walls.

Most of all I felt celebrated − and paid − for the exact thing I had felt so ashamed of: my sexuality.

And so I became anonymous yet finally unmasked. In my personal life I was remote from judgement:

my own or others'. I no longer felt bound by the constraints of a society that hypocritically judged the industry I worked in, yet paid my bills. The gaze – of family, friends, co-workers – suddenly disappeared. I had one-night stands and affairs, men and women, couples, friends, strangers. I felt the world opening like a citrus fruit between my fingers offering me a euphoric mess of tart odors, sweet flesh, sticky juices. Regret became a memory. I explored the limits of my body and mind. Saying yes or saying no. I was hunter and prey. Incrementally discovered I particularly enjoyed being the prey.

The loneliness of living in shadow crept in. Apart from a handful of close friends nobody knew where I was working. The gulf between myself and others was made more acute in their company. I was constantly lying, scared of being caught out. Apart from the occasional boyfriend, I learnt not to tell those I met outside the club. Perhaps in confessing I could have found peace, but I feared the reality of their condemnation and abandonment, which in my mind would do more harm than good.

By then I'd paid off my student loans and debt and felt I had to move on. It wasn't hard to say goodbye to the late nights and pretending this drunk, slobbering guy is just the most fascinating, attractive person you've ever met. I went back to my 'professional' career. Sadly this too involves much pretending the ignorant, ridiculous imbecile you work for is the most fascinating, inspiring person you've ever met.

The story doesn't quite end there. I started dating someone, ironically, who I met the last night I danced at the club. He hated my past, even though he'd met me at the club (I broke my own golden rule, don't mix business and pleasure, and boy was I sorry). I discovered I was the other woman (he had two other girlfriends). His rationale: that because of the number of people I'd slept with, and having been a dancer, nobody would ever marry me. Despite him clearly being a very dirty pot, trash-talking a lovely shiny copper kettle, I believed him. The simple truth is, most people would say the same thing, and have. Though I'm married now, to someone who loves me and knows it all, it still haunts me.

In the struggle to reconcile with my sexual identity I realized I had to make a choice. I could see my past, all the pieces that make up a very intrinsic expression of my sexual self, as socially and morally unacceptable errors in judgement, and either atone for my 'sins', or curl up and die.

Regardless, what do you do with the past? Wrap it tightly and hold it close? There's no colder sheen than the cruel reflection in a listener's eyes. Worse still, left untold... Self-censorship is such an effective cutting tool.

Or – my choice – a radical acceptance. I realized there's nothing more self-affirming than loving yourself for exactly who you are, without judgement.

Through age, and experience, and determination I learned to stand alone, and hell, if you're judging me anyway, how about I just ask for and do what I really want?

THE INS AND OUTS OF VIRGINITY

Katherine

Erstwhile academic, currently unemployed, always gay.

Came of age in the late '90s/early '00s, technically (I grew up with the media and therefore the mentality, of the '30s-'50s) You can find me on Twitter at @CelluloidTears.

My sex life to date reads a little like the punch line to a joke. Well, rather, television and movie characters who are meant to be particularly socially inept are often endowed with a sex life similar to mine, though I think the guys on *The Big Bang Theory* get laid more often than I do. Virginity, for whatever reason, has been turned into something to laugh at. Especially if one is twenty-seven and isn't celibate or otherwise abstaining for any number of accepted, valid reasons (such as religion or health), which, I assure you, I am not. The problem with virginity is, it takes more than one person to change your status and finding an acceptable, willing participant has never been one of my strengths. Such is the peril of being a showtune-loving, drag-queen-emulating, glitter-addicted gay man trapped in a lesbian's body.

I guess most people, especially those who tend toward any form of psychotherapy, would love to attribute my 'repressed' sexuality to my upbringing, which may be partially true, but I hardly think it completely accounts for the way my attitude toward sex ultimately developed. I was raised in a small, suburban city in southeast Wisconsin to parents who married "until death do us part." Divorce in our extended family is relatively rare and always a little shocking. My cousins continually having children is less so. Have you seen *Leave It to Beaver*? My childhood was a little like that, only if the Beaver (ha) had been a girl and June had had a drinking problem. I was raised Catholic, only not like the devout kind, but rather the kind that goes to church on Christmas and Easter. Maybe.

In spite of my cliché upbringing, my parents were almost shockingly progressive for their backgrounds and location. My dad stayed at home with me when I was a baby while my mother worked. My mother kept her maiden name when she married. My parents (and my mother's parents) were incredibly supportive of any extracurricular I showed interest in, whether it was sports, art, theatre, or something fantastically nerdy like film history. Though she did occasionally try to get me into dresses, my mother did, for the most part, allow me to express my gender however I wanted. She's more pleased now that I have grown up to love makeup, jewelry, and glitter, but there were some rough, awkward years in between.

When I was just barely seventeen, quite out of the blue, one day I discovered I was attracted to women. There really hadn't been any hints or clues over the years, it just kind of happened. Where I went to high school, there weren't even whispers of a gay/straight alliance or anything like that. The only whispering that happened was if someone was rumored to be anything other than straight. I hadn't done much (read: any) dating before my revelation, and I did even less after, an aspect of my life that has not changed. Everyone assured me college boys would appreciate me (and I hoped college girls would, too), but college came and went fairly uneventfully, which is a little shocking in and of itself considering I went to a notoriously artsy, liberal-minded, and, frankly, gay college in New York. There were a couple of drunken occasions where making out may have turned into more, but something always held me back. For fun, let's label it Catholic guilt.

After much contemplation, what I've come to realize is that the reason I didn't just 'lose it' in college like so many do is because, for me, it has to mean something. It's not that I don't want to have it (because I do) or am even waiting for *the one* (mostly because I don't believe in 'the one'), it's just, for me, there has to be some something behind it. If I were to find a woman crazy enough to date me for any extended period of time, yes, I would sleep with her. Happily. However, considering it's been the better part of six years since I even made out with someone, I'd say the chances of that happening in the near future are slim to none. C'est la vie.

The weird part about being a twenty-seven-year-old virgin is that you get these virgin superpowers that allow you to see into all the dark corners of your mind that other people get to hide behind clouds of sexual gratification. In the corners of my mind there are abandonment issues and the accompanying trust issues that have allowed me to push pursuing romantic entanglements aside for my career path. Recently, my career path went kaput and with it went the masks for my issues. My issues and lack of time have, in the past, kept me from dating (ever), which has kept me from sex. Honestly, the lack of emotional intimacy bothers me far more than my lack of physical release, particularly because my lack of sex rarely bothers me at all. This fact has puzzled many over the years, as, from what I understand, sex is very enjoyable. Sometimes you can't miss what you never had.

What I think is possibly unique about my own sexual journey is that I didn't have to have sex to go on it. Will I learn more about myself once I start having it? Undoubtedly. But, in the meantime, I continue to grow and learn about myself and my body, in some respects, more thoroughly than people who have a lot of sex. Virgin superpowers, I have them. Also, I'm unemployed and have a lot of time on my hands.

In spite of some of what I've said, I feel the need to assure you, gentle reader, that most days I'm not actually bitter about and have never been embarrassed by being a virgin. I think about sex often, but it's never been a real part of my life, and that doesn't bother me. I don't think it means I know less about my sexuality, either. Without having sex, I can still know what turns me on and what I'm interested in. I can tell you that shower sex sounds dangerous but intriguing. That I've fantasized in public places...and about them. I can tell you that breasts are amazing and that even though I've never done it, I imagine kissing someone you care about must rank pretty high on the Best Feelings Ever list. I don't have to have sex or even the intimacy that leads up to it to know what will work for me. And I certainly don't have to have sex to be comfortable talking about it. I would say the fact that people are generally shocked I'm a virgin speaks to that. Or maybe it's just because no one believes someone can last this long without having sex, who knows.

Yes, I would like to have sex someday, preferably sooner rather than later. But I'm not in a rush. I'd rather it be right than it be right now. I'm stubborn that way.

SEX WORKER MOMMY

Penny Barber

Penny Barber has been a San Francisco-based dominatrix, adult actress, and writer since 2003. She is pansexual, an atheist, an avid reader, lover of animation and also the mother of two brilliant children. Find out more about her at itsmyurls.com/PennyBarber.

I had been working in the adult industry for five years and as a professional switch for three when I found out that I was, well, knocked up. I was unmarried, uninsured, and, though I'm pro-choice, knew with all my heart that I wanted to be a mom.

This had always thrown my coworkers, whether photographers, clients, or fellow adult actresses or dominatrixes, but I have a strong maternal side and love kids. I even worked as an au pair and at a nursery school when still in high school. So who knows? That shy teen you hire to watch your two-year-old may one day be available to spend a little quality time with you!

I didn't think that there was anything incongruous about my desire to breed and my feminism, my desire for raunchy sex and my desire to nurture a child. My boyfriend, now ex-husband, agreed, but I was often met with doubt and disbelief when I said that I wanted to be a mommy. Why on earth would I have chosen to be a sex worker if I wanted kids? Didn't I know that it was inevitable that I would scar my children? That I couldn't do anything but have sex forever and ever? That it was sex or motherhood – not both?

Beyond getting married in a hurry – my conservative Catholic mother has had enough surprises and I wanted to at least give her a legitimate grandchild, which I now realize is an awful reason to get married – I had to decide what I wanted to do with my career. In fact, a lot of us did. Right before I found out that I was expecting, another prominent, local Mistress told me that she had a bun in the oven, and two more pregnancy announcements followed shortly thereafter. It was a kinky baby boom!

It was amazing to have other women to talk to who were experiencing the same confusing, judgemental mess that I was. Most of the dommy mommies I knew had their babies years before they began adult work. They never had to waddle around the dungeon in six-inch stilettos, rushing off to pee every five minutes because a fetus was pushing on their bladders. Speaking of which, pregnancy is great for golden shower scenes!

Out of all the decisions that had to be made, I was always very clear about one thing: one way or another I would keep working. I stopped switching with my clients, but it was better than quitting.

First of all, I worried that I would lose my slot at the gorgeous dungeon I session at, la Maison de la Maîtresse. It's one of the most beautiful venues I've ever seen and is perfectly equipped for the domestic discipline and sissification scenes that I'm so fond of. I was not about to go back to playing in someone's converted garage, thank you very much or, worse yet, cheap motel rooms.

Second, I needed to build up a nest egg for my time off. There are many wonderful things about being a self-employed sex worker, but paid maternity leave is not one of them.

Lastly, my partner wasn't the kinkiest guy on earth. Even if he had been, I thrived on variety, but was not interested in the emotional investment that would accompany finding a personal playmate to keep me busy. Oddly enough, it seemed as though it would be easier for me to wait for men who would pay for the privilege of playing with a pregnant woman than to find one who would do it for free, though I knew it would still be a challenge.

To keep working, I had to build a fetish wardrobe that would encompass my quickly swelling stomach. The other pregnant pro dommes and I frantically searched for lingerie that still looked dominant, trading shopping links and handing down corselets, and I stuffed myself into my leather pants for as long as I could, until they ripped down the back. Eventually I had to settle for a black jersey maternity dress that I wore over and over again. I paired it with the craziest shoes my subs could find to try to make it new for each session. Expensive latex and leather were out of the question and vinyl cracked unbecomingly at even the slightest stretch.

Telling clients of my delicate condition was another hurdle. I lost all my dominant clients overnight. I could no longer be beaten, electrocuted, pierced, or tied in uncomfortable positions. Submissives who had been with me for years expressed concerns over our activities somehow affecting my unborn baby, at least until I informed them that I sure as hell wasn't going to be celibate for the next nine months, so they should enjoy our time together while they could. Others opted to spend hours rubbing my swollen ankles rather than let me click around in my beloved stilettos, but most were simply in awe of the fecund goddess before them.

My breasts, already surgically-enhanced, inflated like balloons. My twenty-four-inch waist grew lush and unrestrained, maxing out at almost fifty inches. My ass plumped and my hips broadened, rendering me a living Venus of Willendorf. I finally had the maternal figure to match my maternal nature and I began attracting more and more clients who wanted to be mothered as well as disciplined. Pregnancy turned me from a thin fetish model with a barely legal schoolgirl look into a voluptuous sex goddess.

I also started doing a lot of cuckold scenes, which was a whole new venue for me to explore. When my first client, a long-term playmate that I still see regularly, asked me to tell him that the baby I was carrying wasn't his, I wasn't sure what he was talking about. The baby *wasn't* his. He'd probably never even seen me completely naked, certainly not in person, anyway. Still, he enjoyed having it rubbed in his face that I was with someone else and I found the idea so amusing that I just went along with it. For those into cuckolding scenes, pregnancy can really drive home the point. The fantasy that a guy would be so hopelessly devoted to me, even when I'm telling him that I'm having my lover's baby and he's just going to have to deal with it, thank you very much, really churns my butter, even if I wouldn't *actually* want to start a family that way.

I kept working until two weeks before my due date, and after that continued working from home, which kept me from going stir crazy as the baby coasted along to two weeks after my due date, only making his grand entrance into the world when my doctor began to plan for induced labor. My new husband tried to get me to stay home sooner, but I felt fine and had been raised on stories of my mother's pregnancy-defying diligence. She worked until the day she had me and was back in the office a week later. I was already planning on taking off a month for post-delivery recovery, which would later turn into six weeks before returning part time. I didn't want to be lazy and a number of my childless clients were just as in need of attention as they ever were. Being a first-time mother, I wasn't sure how to explain to them that I needed time to go to lactation classes or get my things in order or just sleep in preparation for many months of sleepless nights and days with an insomniac baby.

All the time that I continued working around my puffed out belly, adjusting my whipping stance to my new center of gravity and using my now superhumanly thick nails as weapons, I only had one uncomfortable, though thankfully not unsafe, experience with an over-enthusiastic Dutchman.

I don't recall his face exactly, but he was fair, just entering middle age, and slender. He was interested in an adult baby session and arrived with a gift for the baby, a blanket made to look like a flattened lamb. You know the ones I mean: the ones that look a bit like roadkill where the only uncrushed bit is the still-attached head. It was a more or less routine session with one exception: he wouldn't stop touching my belly. I told him to keep his hands off my fundus over and over again, but I finally had to tie his hands down. After the session, he started talking about the different sexual practices in other cultures that involved children. Eventually he started talking about how he thought it should be considered normal for an adult to use his penis as a pacifier for a crying infant. I couldn't get him out of there fast enough.

The next day, he sent an email dripping with compliments and offering to buy me gifts if we could stay in contact. "I felt completely accepted." "The least fear happens when you have done everything that you want in life." "I am happy I met you." I ignored the email and, when he wrote again, I told him simply that I was not interested. Thankfully, he left me – and my baby – alone after that. I thought about reporting him to the police, but was worried about drawing the attention of the police and what that would mean for my child and, in all fairness, talking as he did was not illegal. The services that I provided, however, might be.

Other than that one extremely uncomfortable and creepy experience, my clients were wonderful. Their support was surprising, and gave me a jolt of faith in humanity, which I needed after the Dutchman. Not only did the relationships that I'd built mostly stick, but new clients were just as appreciative of my skills whether or not I was a mom-to-be. Some even went the extra mile, contributing to my children's college funds, shopping around for and purchasing a great diaper bag, remembering my children's birthday with presents, and one went so far as to buy each of my children a beautiful, hand-painted, porcelain box from Tiffany & Co.

Of course, I did lose my best client, S. My experience with S was the closest that I ever came to dating a client. He was very much my type: older, with a full beard and an earring. His circumcised, straight member measured just under nine inches and he came like a bull. He flew to San Francisco from the east coast every few months for long, elaborate sessions and expensive dinners. He always brought gifts, including a bespoke leather collar embossed with my name. He took me to have my navel pierced and paid for the procedure as well as the white gold barbell. Looking up into his eyes as he held me down on the table, his hands pressing my shoulders to the padded leather, as the handsome, young piercer thrust his needle through my flesh, was one of the most intense and erotic experiences of my life.

I told him that I was pregnant with my first child as he was planning a trip out to see me. He'd just taken one, but he liked to start planning them immediately, and considering his almost constant flow of gifts, I didn't mind his desire for extra attention, though I sometimes had trouble keeping up with the lengthy fantasy scenarios that he would write and email to me.

I broke the news to him that I would not be able to

submit to him for almost a year. Also, S had a thing for women under the age of twenty-four who were slender. I knew that even though I was only twenty-three, I was nearing the end of my attractiveness to him and becoming pregnant would probably just age me further in his eyes. His belief that women had an expiration date on their asses kept my relationship with S from becoming anything other than professional, despite our easy back-and-forth, shared interests, and sexual chemistry.

Though he was so tall and imposing, S was extremely shy. I may have been the first person with whom he had ever shared his kinky fantasies, and though I encouraged him to seek out his local community, he preferred to fly across the country to see me – and occasionally my co-worker, Mistress Ren. My pregnancy changed that and he finally became part of his local kink community and started dating kinky women.

He tried to turn his abandonment of me in my time of need into a compliment. "I just can't go nine months without this!" I understood. I had always thought that I was the one who kept him at a distance, that he was more devoted to me than our interactions really warranted, but this reminded me that, while a client may say that he wants to be something more, when reality comes calling, only very few answer. S and I only talked a few times after he moved on. He sent a few gifts for my first son and got a young girlfriend who looked uncannily like me, down to the glasses and strong chin.

After I had figured out how to balance my first child with my career, the second one slid into his place in my life easily and surely. I was the mother I had always wanted to be, while still supporting myself and my little ones as a sex goddess. There were losses along the way and there will be more, but I am experiencing every kind of love that there is, and that makes my life very grand indeed.

UNINTENTIONAL

Kailynn

I am a wannabe celesbian, blogger, educator and a sassily natural ginger working her way through grad school.

I'm twenty-two years old, going on fifty-eight. I have old-fashioned values and, despite my growing up in the '90s and coming of age in the past five to ten years, I've exploded with sexuality in the past few years with the mentality of a fifty-year-old. I can be found at GingerSass.com and @THEGingerSass.

I am a very sexual being. I was a late bloomer (I didn't sleep with anyone until my sophomore year of college), but I certainly indulged in the art of self pleasure during my teen years! My first sexual partner was a girlfriend I had on and off through half of college. We had a very explosive sexual relationship and I spent most of the first year of our relationship exploring all sorts of sexual pleasures with her. I guess you could say, on paper, I'm not very experienced. However, I've tried enough things in the realm of the sex and kink worlds to have a lot more knowledge than most of my friends. I suppose that's why it shocks people when they realize that I've been celibate for over a year.

I didn't set out to spend over a year celibate. The last time I had sex, it was May 25th, 2011. I only remember the date because it was the day after my dog's birthday. Like many episodes of *The L Word*, I was broken up with my ex but still sleeping with her. (Hey, women are complicated - even more complicated when they're dating or attracted to each other.) There was something familiar and sweet about sleeping together that day, but it also proved something to me: I wasn't attracted to her anymore. There wasn't any spark between us, and the sex was mediocre at best. I left her house with an oddly peaceful feeling, and also knowing that whatever was happening between us had to end.

Fast forward to today. I've gone on quite a few dates, but I haven't slept with anyone. A lot of people (and friends) my age seem to find it easy to sleep with new people on a regular basis, but I just can't seem to do that. Past mistakes have helped me to learn that I want to believe that I'm old fashioned. I want to wine and dine for a bit before hitting the sack. I want to have an emotional connection with someone I'm intimate with. I don't want to rush into things. Rushing into things in the past has only led to unhappiness.

My year of unintentional celibacy has taught me the importance of loving myself before loving anyone else. I've reconnected with myself in ways that weren't possible when I was coupled off. For a while, I was even feeling empowered and proud of my body and the curves associated with it. I didn't feel the need to impress anyone with my body. I didn't feel judged and ugly when I gained a few pounds. Would it be a good idea for me to shed a few pounds? Surely, but not for anyone else: for me and my own health.

In an odd turn of events, at the same time that I've gained pride in my body, I've also become ashamed of it. I've recently lost weight from being constantly busy, but I also have a lot of emotional and physical scars from my past that have given me the sense of insecurity I've never experienced before. I have stretch marks that I gained from a bout of illness mixed with depression after a friend's death, and I have a few physical scars from, well, bad decisions and being too caught up in lust to allow myself to be treated well. Despite all this, I'm starting to love myself (as a person) again. Maybe eventually I'll be able to allow myself and others to love my body as well.

I masturbate. A lot. It's become a daily ritual, and, honestly, I don't get as much pleasure from it as I used to. I'm at a sexual low while being at a personal high. I don't worry about what others think of my body because nobody else is seeing it. My blog has let me form connections with brilliant, sexy women who send me free sex toys and queer porn, and that has definitely added to my celibacy. Free toys are very fun ways for rediscovering who you are and what you enjoy.

Celibacy has taught me to take the time to love and appreciate my friends and the small things in life. If a relationship came into my life right now, would I be happy? Sure. Would I give up my celibacy? Probably. Until then, I'm perfectly happy to be celibate and at peace with myself and my vibes.

Plus, I'm saving a lot of money on lube.

INEXPERIENCED, NOT STUPID

Firefly Sub

I'm a thirty-year-old (born in 1982) dog groomer who hates her job, but does it because the money is good and she loves dogs. Had to drop out of college because the government wouldn't give me a loan, and I had a mortgage to pay. I've had to do pretty much anything but what I've wanted to do (like most, I'm sure). I can be found at @Firefly_Sub.

I can't remember a time when I wasn't thinking about sex.

I was about four when I started masturbating. Whenever I would spend the night at my grandmother's house, I would think to myself, "Oh! I can do that thing tonight!" I didn't know what I was doing, not really, but I loved it. I loved the tingly feeling that would explode all over my body.

Growing up an only child, I learned a lot about kissing and other "dirty" things from my best friend and neighbor who had older brothers, and was allowed to watch anything on TV. And I mean anything. I couldn't wait to experience a French kiss, or make out with a boy. I was six, and already dreaming about that one special guy who would turn all of my fantasies into reality.

By the time puberty hit, I had my sexual life mapped out. I planned to lose my virginity around seventeen. I was petrified of pregnancy and STDs, so in my head I knew that the lucky boy would be wearing a condom, and I would be on birth control. You can never be too careful, right?

By the time I actually was seventeen, I was a depressed, suicidal mess with no friends, especially no boyfriends, a mother who had moved away to live in another country, and a broke father who couldn't afford new clothes for me. Not that I ever asked for them. I was an overweight girl in a skinny world. There were no plus size stores in my teenage years, so clothes shopping was a nightmare for me.

At twenty-one, I figured that it would happen sooner or later. Some people are late bloomers. I noticed men looking at me, but I had no self-esteem. And I would have died before making the first move. If no one asked me out, it was fine. Someday my prince would come. I firmly believed it.

Twenty-two came, then twenty-three, twenty-four, twenty-five...

My first kiss happened when I was twenty-four. If

you had told me as a child that I would have to wait twenty-four years for a kiss, I would have laughed in your face. Everyone told me I was pretty. There was no way I would be waiting around like a loser for so long.

My first sexual experience happened last year: my twenty-ninth year on Earth. It was nothing more than kissing, him teasing and pleasuring my breasts, and me cautiously rubbing his penis through his jeans. When he asked me to spend the night, I froze. What was I supposed to do? I liked this guy; I had thought we were just friends. He asked me over to watch a movie, and now he wanted sex? As I was laying on my back looking up at him, I nervously let him know that I was a virgin, and, though I liked him, I wouldn't be having sex with him. At least not that night. He took the news well, and we talked about the whys of my situation, and my nonexistent sexual history. I went home, and I never heard from him again. I would text just to say hi, and nothing. He'd send maybe a word here or there, but no more friendship, no more anything. I didn't know what I had done so wrong, but I wasn't in love with him. I liked him as a friend, so I chalked it up as experience and moved on.

A few months later, I met a man via Twitter who told me I was perfect. He wanted to spend time with me, get to know me. We texted each other constantly, and arranged a meeting on a weekend when I wasn't working. We met for lunch, and he came back with me to my apartment. He had known I was a virgin, and as far as sex goes, we did everything but penetration. He gave me my first experiences with oral, giving and receiving, touching an erect and unclothed penis, fingering, feeling another body pressed against mine while naked. It was eye-opening. I loved it, but I didn't love him. To be honest, I didn't even like him all that much, but I was so desperate to feel.

And I felt like a moron two weeks later when I found out he was married.

I had had my suspicions, but to have it confirmed made me feel like a complete idiot. A couple of weeks later, a new guy I had been texting also turned out to be married as well.

I've become very open about my virginity in the past few months. It is what it is, and I'm not ashamed of it. It's the responses that I can't stand. The ones that I hate are the responses from women. They look at me like a freak. Tell me that they can "get me popped." Look at me in pity. My favorite line I've gotten was, "I wish I was still a virgin." I looked at her in disbelief and said, "No, you don't."

The men have a completely different reaction. I will never hear from them again, or they become fascinated by me. It's like they see my hymen as a novelty, a prize that they can win.

I've had more men than I can remember tell me they want to be my first. If I was naïve and twenty, I would be honored. I would feel so wanted and amazing. But as I'm a virgin at thirty, I see life a little differently.

I'm not a stupid girl, but I am inexperienced. People seem to get the two very confused.

I hate my virginity. It makes me frustrated. I hate that I can't go out and find someone for a one night stand because this membrane and my paralyzing fear of the first time pain is in my way of pleasure. I hate that people look at me differently when they find out. I hate that most people my age are married, and having children, and I've never even had a boyfriend. I hate that men a couple years older than me are becoming tired of their marriages, and are looking for fun, and I'm there. I'm available, and I'm offering something they haven't had in a long time, if ever. I hate the women who think they're helping by offering me a man who will fuck me. I hate even more the women who look at me with pity in their eyes. I hate the feeling that I'm disappointing my mother. She was married and pregnant with me at my age, and though I've never wanted that in my life, I feel like I'm doing so many things wrong.

I know it will happen someday, but it's been hard realizing that my prince isn't on his way. My prince is probably out there married to another woman who hasn't led a life governed by fear.

At Least We Tried

Alicia Wolfe

Wine connoisseur with an amazing rack and a dog of an ex-husband. She leads a pretty normal life as a number cruncher, wife and mom/slave to three cats.

A former BFF (geography and life experience have caused us to drift apart a bit) and I used to discuss sexuality on a fairly regular basis. There were several reasons for this:

- We were both married to army men. Our

men were not homophobic themselves, but the issue seemed to come up a lot in that crowd.

- We both have nice racks. Seriously, on New Year's Eve several of the aforementioned army men (to whom we were not married) paid us to flash our boobs. We all agreed it was both money well-spent and well-earned.

- The subject is simply fascinating.

It was her idea to view it as a spectrum and I quickly saw she was right. Most people are somewhere on either end of the spectrum: either solidly homosexual or solidly heterosexual. And there are the bisexuals smack in the middle. We came to the conclusion, however, that women tend to be closer to the center than men. We are simply more open to experimentation within our own sex.

Perhaps it's because breasts are beautiful and penises are...not so much. I am heterosexual, but I really appreciate a nice rack.

All these discussions also revealed a secret: she wasn't sure if she had ever had an orgasm. Now, we all know that anyone who isn't sure about it definitely *hasn't*, so I took her to the toy store and helped her pick out her first vibrator.

It turns out I was right. She hadn't ever had an

orgasm before. It took a vibrator, not a man, for her to learn that.

And so, when our husbands were deployed, and mine wanted a divorce, and hers sent her some bizarre letter from halfway around the world about how he wasn't sure if he wanted to continue the marriage, we experimented.

We were drunk and emotional about our respective husbands and thought that maybe everything would just be easier if we ditched men all together and made our own couple. We were both sex-starved with no men around and she had only recently discovered how enjoyable it could be.

So one night it just happened.

It was kind of like my first time all over again in some ways. The lights were definitely *off*. We were completely under the covers. There was a fair amount of fumbling around.

But kissing is easily transferable and we were both rather excited. I spent a lot of time kissing, nuzzling and sucking those glorious boobies of hers while I fingered her. As enjoyable as it all was, I just couldn't bring myself to go downtown.

But that didn't stop her from trying it on me.

It was very enjoyable at first. Probably because we were so sex-starved. And attention-starved. Everything felt *so* good at first. But after a little while it just...fizzled. For both of us. It turns out that neither of us was as far to the middle of that spectrum as we previously thought.

But hey, at least we tried.

SCHOOLED

Taffy Davenport

I am a newly separated after twenty years of marriage. I have been a stay-at-home mom for most of sixteen years and have just started working in the last year. I love to write erotica.

I was born in 1972 and married when I turned eighteen to a man nine years older than myself. I write at SmutByMissJane.com.

This story was painful to write, but I believe putting it

down on paper was therapeutic.

I was going back to school. Human services. I wanted to be an advocate for people with disabilities, or something similar. I had started school before but had to quit due to issues with childcare for my daughter. This time I was more confident. I had just gotten back together with my husband after an almost two-year split, I had lost 40lbs. and I was going to the gym at least five days a week. Everything seemed right in the world. A new beginning.

In two of my classes there was a man named James. He was well over six feet tall and was quite the flirt. I sat in front of him in our counseling class and when we had to pair up to practice our counseling skills he and I would sometimes pair up.

He would flirt with me and I would blush and act all silly like no one had ever flirted with me before.

My husband worked two jobs at the time: his day job installing windows and doors and his night job helping a friend remodel his home. I saw him very little. When I did see him I told him about James. I was like a giddy little girl telling my husband about this guy who was flirting with me. He just listened with a grin on his face. He was not the jealous kind. It seemed like he thought he had to be happy for me because I liked the attention.

The flirting got more and more serious. Instead of it just being some little compliment or some joke that would make me blush it started being a bit more about sex: asking me personal questions about my sex life with my husband or asking about what I had experienced in the past.

I started looking for him in the cafeteria when I got to school and would sit with him until it was time for class. I started dressing up for school. I'd wear things like a blouse instead of a t-shirt, a tight denim skirt with lacy white knee high socks and black platform heels. Of course I'd do my hair and makeup as well. I had already been dressing up more and more due to the weight loss and the fact that I was feeling pretty hot with this new body of mine.

One day James asked me for a ride home. He lived in the same part of the city that I did. He lived in the drug and alcohol treatment part of the veterans center, across from the hospital. He flirted with me all the way there and talked about how he would like to have sex with me. I blushed and never knew what to say but would say things like "James, you know I'm married" while smiling from ear to ear. He would tell me that he wasn't trying to date me, that he just wanted to have sex with me. When I would blush or act coy he would tell me that I was too old to be embarrassed by the things he said. I told him that I had been married since I was eighteen.

I went home and told my husband about giving him a ride home. He casually told me that I should stay away from this guy because I might be enjoying the flirting but this guy was serious about getting into my pants. I sometimes found myself wishing that my husband would get mad and forbid me to ever speak to James again.

I continued to flirt with James. I enjoyed the attention too much and didn't want to give that up. I had always practiced living in the moment and rarely thought of the repercussions.

The next time he asked me for a ride I heard him tell our teacher that he was sick and that another student (me) had agreed to drive him home. I felt a bit uneasy about it, but I didn't want to say no. I didn't want him to stop flirting. I wanted him to like me.

When we pulled out of the parking ramp he slid his hand up my leg and pulled my skirt up a bit. I pulled it back down and blushed and told him to stop, however I said it in the I'm-only-saying-this-because-I-don't-want-to-seem-like-a-whore kind of way. I had a whole list of reasons why I shouldn't have sex with him, apart from the fact that I was married. Most of the things on the list were things that I always worried about: being self-conscious about my body, things like that. I even told him some of those things. He had an answer for everything. He said I didn't have to be self-conscious about my body because he'd just pull up my skirt and take off my panties. I'd blush again and look away, but I was filing away all the things he said. I think I used them later on when I was going through the pros and cons in my head. I honestly think I worried more about if James would like me and if I could go through with it than I worried about my husband and whether he would leave me or not.

When I got almost to the veterans center I told him "Yes. Yes I'll have sex with you." He said "Ok" and smiled but didn't seem all that shocked about it. I asked him about condoms. He made some crack about how he doesn't just carry them around in his wallet. I told him we could stop at the pharmacy and he could run in.

I waited in the car in front of the pharmacy. When he came out he appeared to put something in his pocket but he had no bag. When he got in the car I asked him if he got the condoms and he said yes. I thought it was a little odd that there was no bag but I figured he wouldn't lie about something that I would soon find out about anyway.

There was a motel on the side of the road and he directed me to pull in there. I was not that excited about it being one of those old motels where all the entrances to the rooms were on the outside and to get to the second floor you had to climb the outside wooden stairs to get up to the balcony.

I waited outside while he went into the little office and paid for the room. When he came out he complained about the cost of the room as he walked toward me. He couldn't believe that he had to pay $49 for a single room.

He opened the door to the room and I stepped in. He quickly took his shoes and clothes off and got into bed.

I remember exactly what I was wearing that day. A black sleeveless shirt, a black A-line skirt with a bit of a ruffle at the bottom, white knee socks and calf high black boots with three-inch heels and a buckle on the side. I removed my boots and quickly got under the covers with all my clothes on. I remember when I was getting into the bed I noticed several pieces of grey duct tape on the wall, right by my head. It looked like it was covering up a big hole in the wall.

I laid down facing him, with my hand under my head, propped up on my elbow. He asked me what I wanted to do. I said "Can we talk for a little while first?" I was nervous and was hoping we would take things slow. He didn't respond to what I said unless you count immediately kissing me a response.

After he kissed me for a few seconds, and before I knew what was happening, he was on top of me. This more than six-foot tall man on top of this five-foot tall girl. He quickly reached under my skirt and pulled my panties down and off. He was instantly inside of me. I felt kind of like I was in outer space. All these things were happening so fast and I didn't feel like I had control over any of them. He raised my feet over my head and was having sex with me. I just laid there, still. I noticed that my breathing started getting heavy and I started to feel like I couldn't get my breath. I said to him "wait! wait!" and I put my hand up a little bit in a stopping motion. He either didn't hear me or he didn't want to hear me. He continued on and I decided it was important that I just go along with things. I didn't want to say "stop!" in some loud voice and have him ignore me again. I figured doing nothing was better than this turning into a horribly ugly scene. It finally dawned on me that I was just lying there so when he laid on top of me, with his face near mine, I wrapped my arms around his back and moved them around to act like I was participating. I didn't want him to think I was a dead fuck. I think I started making some faint noises as well. He was not well endowed at all, thankfully, so there was no discomfort whatsoever. He took a lot longer than I thought he would. I couldn't wait for it to be over. Finally there was the last few, and harder, thrusts. It felt all wet all of a sudden so I asked "did you just cum inside of me?" He said "yep."

He laid down next to me, on his back. I asked him why he didn't use a condom? He replied "I don't use condoms. I hate them." I asked him if he even bought condoms at the pharmacy. "Nope." I didn't respond. He got up and went to the bathroom. I waited and then went in after him. The bathroom was dark and had a little shower stall in the corner. The toilet was next to the small sink that hung on the wall. There was a small mirror over the sink.

We made lunch plans after that. I took him to a lunch place where my husband and daughter and I went to breakfast sometimes. He complained about how the food was weird and the chicken was dry, but he still picked up the check. I did my best to be charming and not say too much to disrupt anything. After all I still wanted him to like me.

I was flying high for a couple days afterward feeling like I was something special because I was able to have casual sex like everyone else. After a couple of days reality set in and I broke down and told my husband everything. He was mad and hurt but still comforted me while I cried because of how bad I felt. I'm not sure if I felt worse because I cheated on my husband or because James never liked me as much as I wanted him to.

On my husband's request I started seeing a therapist, and started going to a support group as well. He said that I could stay in school if I thought I could stay away from James. I quit going.

For almost two years afterward I replayed that whole scenario with James in my head several times a day. Thinking about what I could have done differently. At what point should I have walked away. Why I did it. I had a loving husband, but was I lonely anyway? Did I need or want attention so badly that I was willing to do anything for it? Did I think so little of myself? My husband? Our daughter? Things improved with time and life went on. I don't think my husband ever looked at me the same way he had before I cheated and I don't think he ever completely trusted me again. I still don't really know why I did it. There were many theories tossed around by the therapist and the people at the support group, but there was never a consensus. I gave up trying to figure out why I would do such a thing.

What I do know is that I will never do anything like that again. It's not like the movies where affairs are glamorous and romantic, taking place in five-star hotels, making love for hours, then cuddling, talking, and ordering room service afterward. I think I believed it would be some version of that, or at least I wanted it to be. I learned a hard lesson. I hurt myself that day, as well as my husband. That hurt continued long after.

JUST A GOOD SOUTHERN GIRL

Sweet Cheeks

Just a simple southern housewife with a naughty side.

I'm convinced that almost every girl I know has in some way or another experimented with another girl at least once and most of those who insist they never did are lying. At the same time it's become a huge source of shame and guilt for me as an adult, the kind I hope my daughter never experiences. Thank you religious, southern upbringing! It's not something I've ever told anyone about but I always wonder if the people involved early on think I'm a deviant even though they were just as 'guilty'. I secretly went through phases where I thought I was bi but I always knew I could never be in a relationship with a girl beyond close friendship. My need for the (perceived) security of being with a man is too strong. I don't necessarily totally regret my own experiences, they've helped shape me into one of those people who make the phrase "it's always the quiet ones" so very true.

My first sexual experience of any sort was at a sleepover with two friends in fifth grade. They wanted to role play different scenarios as a married couple and it was apparent they had done that before. I don't remember much aside from some kissing and touching but not directly 'down there'. I enjoyed it immensely and couldn't wait to play like that again. Sometime after that one of the girls spent the night at my house. While lying in my bed we decided to pretend we were married. We kissed, touched, and pretended to hump each other. Then she put her hand down my panties and touched me 'there'. Right then I had my first ever orgasm. I would spend the next few years trying unsuccessfully to recreate that feeling myself.

A new friend moved down the street later that year and I was pleased when she suggested we practice kissing. Kissing and humping while we took turns wearing a balled up pair of socks down our pants became commonplace for us but I never had an orgasm. She claimed to but I was never certain we really knew enough to know for sure.

I would later go on to fool around with a good friend in junior high. She was more experienced than me but I had a serious boyfriend and welcomed the practice. I loved for her to suck on my tits and enjoyed fingering her. Once she suggested I go down on her but I had no idea how that was done so I laughed it off. Once in high school we had little contact and she dropped out. We reconnected after I was in college and one time she asked me if that was just a phase. "Of course!" I'd answer, not wanting anyone to ever think I was really into that.

By high school I was more interested in meeting guys, getting a date, and actually making out than I was in just practicing with friends. It would be after I had a serious boyfriend and was in college before I'd feel any further interest in fooling around with girls again. My studies were focused on feminist theory and I was quite liberal. It was nice to see a girl and wonder what it would be like to make out with her but I was way too shy to ever act on this. During my junior year an older girl in one of my classes stopped because she recognized the homework I was doing. The following semester she was in my gay & lesbian literature class (cliché, I know). I'd secretly hoped I'd find someone in this class to hook up with but never thought it'd be her. She was in a relationship and living with another girl. We started talking and went out a few times, knowing where things were headed. One night we'd been out to a gay bar and started kissing. She lived nearby and her girlfriend would be working until really late so we quickly went to her house. I must admit that the feeling of having a girl go down on you for the first time is incredible. That memory has remained part of my somewhat limited 'spank bank'. I would eventually have the pleasure of successfully going down on her. Making a lesbian come felt victorious to me. Once (I'm not sure why not more) she fucked me with a strap-on. I've recently started wishing I'd had the chance to do the same. Our fling ended after about six months, she felt guilty and I didn't want to be a factor in the breakup with her girlfriend.

After that I'd hope to hook up with other girls but was way too shy to ever make my thoughts known. That part of me just faded away along with my idealism after I completed my feminist theory coursework. I'd dabble again if I knew no one would find out. Even now, as asexual as my life as a minivan-driving, Christian-preschool-volunteering stay-at-home mom has become, I'd be thrilled if any of my friends made a move on me.

THEN AND NOW

Tizz Wall

Tizz Wall is the irreverent Jane-of-all-trades, taking on the world with leather and lace. She is a California-certified domestic violence counselor and sex educator. She works one million and one jobs (pro-domme, writer, speaker, odd-gig-taker) and lives in Oakland, California. You can read more about her at about.me/tizzwall.

THEN

We were under the bed, hidden from the light, and

Jamie told me she had a new game for us to play. "Pull down your pants," she told me. Ignoring my refusal, she pulled them down herself. Jamie was always in control. The memory becomes obscure after this, stripped down to the view of the coils under the mattress and the sound of her voice. Her mother called for us, and we scrambled, filled with worry and guilt, caught with our hands in the cookie jar. Her hand, rather. She hastily rolled out from under the bed, and yelled at me to do the same.

At three, my mother found blood in my underwear. Years later, the story was told that my cherry was popped while riding a bike. Somehow, that sounded better than being forcefully fingered by another child.

I had sex for the first time with my first boyfriend. I had been sneaking on to the porch for make-out sessions in the balmy Sacramento heat every other night of the summer. He had been pushing for us to have sex, and each time, the pressure grew in intensity. We had met when I was ten and he was fifteen, but years had passed. There were no particular illusions about my virginity being some sort of flowery treasure to withhold, but I knew that I wanted to be in love with the first person I slept with. He had been telling me how beautiful I was, and how much he was in love with me for months, but I couldn't bear saying it back. It made me uncomfortable. Being too young to understand how to process such profuse and incessant expressions of affection, I was instead awkward, uncomfortable, uneasy. It wasn't until the fall, when mornings became full of hot tea and frost-covered grass, that I realized I loved him too.

I ditched class to go to the clinic to get birth control, and sat him down to tell him that I would be getting an abortion if I got pregnant. I told him thirteen was too young to be having a baby. He nodded along and agreed. After all, what hot-blooded seventeen-year-old boy is going to say no based on such stipulations? We had sex at the end of the bed. It was over quickly and I remember thinking, "That's it? That's what all the hype was about?" He laid on top of me, breathing heavily, and I said aloud, almost to myself, "Oh, we can do better than that!" He leaned up on his arms, moving frantically, and with a quiver of insecurity asked, "What?" I couldn't bear to tell him that it wasn't as good for me as it was for him.

He had gone down on me already, and had even gotten a tongue piercing to improve the experience. He stood at my front door, showing me his swollen tongue and waving at my mother. I wasn't yet ready to return the favor. I convinced myself that maybe if I tried it, I would get turned on. Already I knew that most fears could be overcome by unabashed boldness, and concluded this would be the case.

Once, in the dark of my room, we started. I sat on

his legs and put his penis in my mouth. I sat up, a stone of discomfort in the pit of my stomach, and he begged me not to stop. I told him how much I didn't want to anymore, but he put his hands on my elbows, begging me to continue. I said to him, "B, I can't. Please, let's just stop," and moved to get off of his legs. His arms, thick with teenage muscle from playing football and getting in street fights, held me in place.

"Please, please don't stop," he said.

"Please, B. I just don't want to anymore."

"Just a little bit more. Don't stop."

He wouldn't let me move until I continued. After that I didn't want to have sex anymore. We dated for another eight months, but the memories are blurry at best. Strangers rape people. Crazy people rape people. People who want to hurt women will rape them, but people you love (and who love you) don't want to hurt you, so they would never do such things. It couldn't be that.

*****

The following January, it snowed in the valley for the first time in over ten years. I am never entirely sure what constitutes a miracle. I have never been sure of what love is supposed to look like.

"Oh, did your cat do those?" Melissa responded to the question with a sneer, glancing down at the jagged marks across her wrists. The freshest lines were scabs, bright red and swollen around the edges, and beneath them there was another layer of faded scars. She rolled her eyes and muttered, "Uh, yeah. My cat. That's it."

She glanced over at me, and when our eyes met, there was a moment of mutual understanding. Everyone who is part of the 'Fucked Up Kid' crew knows the subtle exchanges that serve as membership cards. One of the first lessons in a childhood filled with vicious outbursts and misdirected vitriol is in learning to read subtext. You learn how eyes communicated love, or regret, or violence. You learn what it means to fight or flee. You learn how to dissect intellectual armor and brokenhearted poker faces.

The ponytail of the girl who had asked the initial question bobbed as she yammered on about her cat, but we had stopped listening. Melissa still hadn't taken her eyes off of mine. She knew that I knew that those cuts weren't from the paw of a fuzzy creature. From that moment, at camp, we became friends. She was fourteen, three years older than me, and absolutely, undeniably the first girl I wanted. The shivers of graceless teenage adoration shot through me. Melissa, with her shaved head and sliced arms and torn jeans, is burned into my brain, leaving my head spinning with memories of tingling pubescent lust and confusion.

NOW

He pushes me against the wall, our mouths pressed and open to each other. My left leg is curling up around his right, starting to wrap around him, and he presses his body against mine. He pulls away as quickly as he pushed against me, grabs my hand, and leads me into the living room. He kisses me again, and sits back on the couch.

"I want you so fucking bad right now," I tell him, my voice low. I straddle him on the couch, pressing my chest to his.

"Oh, really?" He smirks and put his hands through my short, dark hair, pulling my head back. As I lean back, he looks me in the eyes. Arousal. Amusement. The air is heady, and our game has started. He slaps me across the face; instantly, a tingling sensation rushes through my entire body. We do this power play back and forth all the time, and although the pain is always more intense than I remember it, the pleasure that fills me is equally strong. He softly touches my cheek, running his hands up my face, to my ear, and back down my neck. He takes his time with this part, building anticipation and countering the harsh hits with soft caresses. I flinch and stare at his face. It may be strange to call a man beautiful, but the power and desire in his face make this already good-looking man gorgeous.

He laughs.

"Are you okay?"

I nod, struggling to form words at this point. All I can manage is "Don't stop."

He slaps me again this time. Harder. My cunt is wet. He loosens his hold on my hair and I rush my mouth toward his. The soft warmth of his kiss is broken by him biting my lip, causing me to cry out. The rush continues throughout my body in waves, unabated, both pleasure and pain and pleasure and pain.

He takes me, with bites and slaps and orders. He takes me in a way that may seem non-consensual, but this is what I want. This is what we talked about. I can barely contain myself as he fucks me with equal parts brutality and affection. He pulls back momentarily, and I beg him to choke me again. Please, don't stop.

This is what I wanted. This is what I asked for. What was forcibly delivered, the acts that left lasting charred marks around the vulnerable parts of my soul, was now something I begged for. What does that make me?

This isn't making love; we aren't in love, but the affection is undeniable. At the end, his semen paints itself across my chest, and we lay together and laugh. He rubs my neck and kisses me on the forehead. We fall asleep, limbs entwined and akimbo.

*****

I took a gulp of wine and I said to Jen, "But I don't feel queer enough since I haven't been in a real queer relationship. I have only been in relationships with men. And now that I finally feel ready to call myself 'queer', to openly pursue that queerdom, I am getting involved with this guy."

Jen shook her head at me, and put her wine glass down.

"That is such bullshit. That is totally internalized misogyny. You are queer if you say you are queer, and if you feel queer. We are not defined by the people we are fucking. That is complete bullshit, and you know it. You are not defined by the person you are with."

Truth from such admirable friends can make a hard heart soften and grow. Blue eyes, wide like windows, welled up with tears.

"You are not defined by the person you are with."

ARE WE DOING THIS WRONG?

Hipster Homemaker

The Hipster Homemaker is a late-twenty-something wife, mother, childbirth educator, birth doula, and lover of life. When she's not busy navigating the world of AP parenting or teaching expectant mothers about the birth process, she enjoys cooking, knitting, yoga, wine, and bad television.

From the outside looking in, I seem every bit the 'good girl.' I always got good grades, never got in trouble, and never got caught with my panties down. In high school, I had a good number of boyfriends, all of which I refused to sleep with. I am far from religious, and certainly not put off by sexuality, but as a young girl in high school, sex seemed to have too many negative consequences for me to want to do it. Sure, there were times I *wanted* to, but I always held back. Looking back, I also really got off on the power of telling these guys "no" when they wanted to move things along. Nope, I'm not going to fuck you. Too bad, dude, move on.

Freshman year of college, however, I met the man who eventually became my husband (and father of our two-year-old-son). I was nineteen, and ready to rid myself of my virgin status. So was he. Plus, I really *liked him*. Like, A LOT more than any of the other guys I had dated. So, after a few weeks of dating, we had sex. It wasn't awesome. We were both first-timers and didn't have any idea what we were doing, or what we liked. I swear, I honestly thought we just did it *wrong*. Like, maybe we didn't actually have sex after all. So, we talked about it. We read about it. We tried different things. Pretty soon, we were *really good.*

Now, when I tell people that my list of sexual partners consists of my marriage license, I inevitably get the following questions or comments: "Oh, you were waiting until marriage?" or "You just think it's good because you don't have anything else to compare it to." No, we did not wait until we were married. We waited about three weeks. We didn't get married for another five-and-a-half years. And no, I don't just think it's good because I haven't slept with anyone else. I *know* it's good. And here's why:

As cliché and dorky as this sounds, we really, really cared about each other and wanted to please each other. We also did a lot of research. We read sex books and magazines together. We talked about what we wanted to try and what we didn't. Then, afterwards, we would go over our new adventure, move by move, and talk about what felt good, what didn't, what we wanted more/less of, and how we could do better next time. Many nights, 'next time' was about twenty minutes later. We were young, horny, and couldn't get enough of each other.

Later, I got a job doing sex toy parties to help pay for college. When you can get any toy you want at cost, things definitely spice up in the bedroom. Not only did it make our time together a lot more fun, but the experimentation I was doing on my own also led me to find things I liked that we could do as a couple, as well.

I have found that since we are (and have always been) so comfortable and open with each other, our sex life reflects that. We are never afraid to try new things, talk about what works, what doesn't and what our limits are.

We occasionally do roleplaying. I do not like to be in a submissive position at all, so even if my role is traditionally the submissive, I always flip it, and end up being the dom. Our favorite scenarios are police officer and naughty girl getting pulled over (who is really, really bad, and will do anything to get out of another ticket!), professor/student, strangers having a one night stand (and don't know each other's names), oh, and of course, the cheerleader effect: dress up like a cheerleader and your man is putty in your hands. "Coach, you *can't* kick me off the team! Take off your pants and I'll show you why..."

I also enjoy being very dominant and restraining him in various ways. Tying him up, handcuffing him to the bed (or coffee table, or dresser!), blindfolding him, spanking him, etc. To me, nothing gets me hotter than seeing my husband, who is the size of your average NBA player, being rendered completely helpless by a girl who is 5'3" on a good day. We do engage is some light cuckolding, in which I tell my husband that there is no way he is going to be able to get me off and his technique just isn't up to my standards. He has to prove himself a worthy lover.

Then, there's the dirty talk. I can't remember the last time we had sex and dirty talk *wasn't* involved. I constantly had a filthy monologue running in my head, but was always afraid to say those things out loud. Finally, one day, I let it loose. Roleplaying was a good outlet for me to get started with dirty talk, because it wasn't 'me' saying those things, it was my 'character'. Eventually, though, I just started blurting out whatever nasty thought was in my head. And I never stopped.

Truth be told, not all of these scenarios always end well. There are times when one (or both) of us will burst out laughing from something the other says or does. Sometimes, things that seem hot in a porno or in a book don't feel that great in real life. But, we keep trying new things. After nine years together, and a 9lb. baby tumbling out of my vagina, my husband still wants to have wild sex with me. And I with him. Even with a two-year-old banging on the door.

So, although I may not have a lot of notches on my bedpost, I sure as hell can rock it off the frame.

THE FIRST NIGHT

Lynn Lacroix

I'm pretty much your typical suburban wife. I'm the woman you wave to in church every Sunday and the woman you meet in the grocery store wearing sweats and trying to find the best deals on groceries. But I have another side. It's a side that very few people know about. I'm a submissive.

I was raised in a great family. I had a great childhood. I was a good church-going, white bread American girl. I lost my virginity the first time I ever got drunk at age eighteen. That opened up a whole new side of my personality. I found out how much I love sex. I wanted more. I immediately realized that I fell into the submissive category. BDSM porn was the only kind that ever turned me on, and I only really wanted to be with men who had a dominant air about them.

Although I had several fun, kinky boyfriends in college, I married the first and only man who has ever given me an orgasm. He doesn't share my kinky side, but he indulges me when I ask. To make up for some of that part of myself that I feel like I'm lacking I write erotica. Specifically, BDSM erotica. Despite this side of me, I really am an average woman and I think there are a lot more like me.

This is one of my stories.

I am nervously waiting at the bar of the hotel where we agreed to meet. I am wearing a black, slinky dress with nothing underneath and patent leather pumps; just as he instructed me. Thank god my boobs haven't started to sag yet and I can get away without wearing a bra unless it is really cold. I look younger than my thirty-one years. I am thin, but have naturally full hips and breasts. My hair is straight and brown. My eyes are hazel. I have a very clear complexion and rarely wear makeup (tonight being an exception). I nervously sip my cosmo, stare at the clock, and start to wonder if he is really coming.

*****

Let me take you back a few weeks. I got a little

tipsy one night and did something I've always wanted to. I put a profile on an adult website. I filled out the basics. Name: Olivia (I don't know why I used my real name), Age: thirty-one, Relationship Status: single. I posted a picture of myself from my vacation in the Bahamas three months ago. In it I am wearing a bikini that leaves very little to the imagination. Then I got to the About Me section. I wasn't really sure what to put, so I wrote: "I think I'm submissive." That's it. Just those four little words.

Over the next couple of days I got a few messages, but one stuck out. It was from a man named Grant. All his message said was that I sounded like I was 'trying to find my true self' and he gave me a telephone number to call. It took me a full day of doubting and nail-biting to pick up the phone and make the call.

"Hello?" says a deep, obviously male voice.

"Um. Hi. Is this Grant?" I ask.

"Yes. What can I do for you?"

"This is Olivia," I say.

"Oh. Hello Olivia. In that case you will from here on out refer to me as Sir. Do you understand?"

"Yes. Um. I mean, yes Sir."

We start out talking about me, my life, and my

previous sexual experiences. Grant asks a lot of questions. Some are really hard to answer. Then the conversation turns to him. Grant is thirty-five, works as an architect, and loves to play basketball on the weekends. I learn that Grant is an experienced Dom. He has had many casual BDSM encounters and a few D/s relationships. He is looking for the right submissive for a long term relationship. He says that he is intrigued by my lack of experience, that he loves training new submissives.

Grant asks me to send him porn images that I like. I do. The usual stuff: a woman tied up and blindfolded, another of a woman tied down and being fucked by a man with bulging muscles. Once I send him those images he begins to tell me stories. He tells me stories of encounters he has had with various women. Then he starts telling me in great detail what he wants to do with me. The rough but eager sound of his voice coupled with the things that he is saying make me want to pull out my vibrator while we are still on the phone, but Grant tells me that I am not to masturbate unless he instructs me too.

We carry on like this for a week and a half before we agree to meet at a posh hotel in the city. He tells me what to wear, what time to be there, and where to wait for him. He is very specific and makes it very clear that there will be consequences if I don't follow his orders to the letter.

*****

Back to the present. Just as I start to think that the whole thing was some twisted joke and that Grant isn't coming I feel a hand wrap around my waist and a familiar voice say, "Hello Olivia." I turn around to see a handsome, very tall man. He has to be at least 6'4. He has sandy blonde hair that looks like it probably curls naturally but he keeps it cut and styled so that it never really can. He has beautiful blue eyes. I can't tell much about his physique due to him being dressed in a suit other than that he is height-weight proportionate and appears to be muscular.

Before I can say anything Grant firms his grip on my waist, pulling me to my feet and leaning down to kiss me. His mouth is so hot it feels like it is on fire. He eagerly kisses my lips and parts them with his tongue. His tongue explores my mouth with more expertise than any other man I have ever kissed. My knees start to feel like Jell-O. At this point, Grant is having to hold me up by my waist. He pulls his mouth away from mine and says with a wicked grin, "The room is all ready. Shall we?" All I can do is nod in the affirmative. "Answer me. Now!" "Yes, Sir." I barely croak out. Oh god, I am not making a very good first impression. Grant would think I was a mute if we hadn't had all those nights of talking on the phone.

I am regaining my composure as Grant leads me to the elevator. We get into the elevator and Grant presses the button for the seventh floor. We get to our floor, then to our room. Grant unlocks to the door and leads me inside. I can tell that he has already been up here. There is a duffle bag on the desk and a glass of whiskey on the rocks next to it. Grant can sense my nervousness.

He smiles at me and says, "I am so glad to finally meet you Olivia. You look beautiful. Don't be nervous. I'm not going to do anything that you don't want me to. Remember your safe word. Do you remember it?"

"Yes Sir. It is 'mercy,'" I answer.

"Good girl. Now step back so I can get a good look at you. Damn, you are gorgeous. Take off that dress so I can see if you followed my instructions."

I slide the straps of my dress off of my shoulders and let it fall to the floor as Grant takes off his suit jacket and tie, and loosens his collar and sleeves. He smiles when he looks at my naked body.

"Perfect." This affirmation makes me smile and puts me even more at ease. It is confusing to me why I want to please this man so badly. I mean, this is the first time we've even met.

"Get on your knees. Eyes lowered. Don't speak unless I tell you to." Grant says in a firm, but not angry tone. I immediately drop to my knees and lower my gaze to the floor.

"Olivia, tell me why you are here with me now," he says.

"I am here because I want you to dominate me, to teach me how to be submissive." I answer with a shaky voice.

"Very good. Tonight, I own you completely. Your body is mine to do with what I wish. This is about me, not you. However, you will love it. You will beg me for more and if you are good I might just reward you with what you want. Now, I want you to stand up and go over to the bed. Put your hands on the edge of the bed and your ass in the air."

I do as I'm told but I am shaking. It isn't from fear though, it's anticipation and desire. There is something about this man that makes me want to give into him completely. Grant takes his shirt off. I sneak a peek by looking over my shoulder and can see that he is very well built. His muscles are well toned and he is obviously very strong. I quickly look away and back at the bed.

"I saw that." Grant says. "I was going to go easy on you this first time, but now you've broken the rules and need to be punished. I want you to count. You will receive thirty strokes." He quickly smacks the left side of my ass with his hand. It stings and I am taken aback.

"Ouch! One!" He brings his hand down on the right side.

"Two!" This continues for thirteen more strokes until my ass is burning all over, but my body betrays the pain. My pussy is soaking wet. He has stopped. What is going on? He said thirty and that was only fifteen. I don't have to wonder for long. I hear something whizz through the air and then something thin and stinging lands on my ass. He is using a riding crop now. I guess he had one in that duffle bag.

"Ah! Sixteen!" I gasp. He brings it down again.

"Seventeen!" I hear the crop whizz through the air again and I brace myself, but nothing happens. Grant laughs a wicked little laugh. Then he slaps my ass again with the crop.

"Eighteen!" There are tears welling up in my eyes now. Not really from the pain (though that is significant) but more from the sense of release that I am experiencing. I feel like I've needed this all along. The cropping continues until we reach thirty and Grant stops. I am nearly sobbing at this point. Grant rubs my sore ass with his strong hands. He picks me up and lays me on the bed.

"Are you okay?" He asks. I nod. He kisses me tenderly on my forehead and then on my lips. He wraps his arms around me and continues kissing me while I recover. The emotional release that he has just given me makes me want him even more. I cling to him while he is holding me and eagerly kiss him back.

"Lay back." He says. I slide to the head of the bed and lie on my back. He goes over to the duffle bag. He retrieves two satin ties. He uses them to bind my wrists to the posts of the bed. Then, he goes to the foot of the bed and bends down between my legs. He kisses my thigh. The kisses get higher, getting closer and closer to my pussy. I feel his wet, hot tongue circling my clit. He is teasing me. I moan.

Grant licks up all the wetness that his spanking created. He slides his tongue into my pussy and rubs my clit with his nose. I am so close to coming. I can feel it building inside me when he stops. He slowly kisses his way up my stomach, my breasts, my neck, and finally he gets to my mouth. This kiss is the most intense we have shared. I can taste my own body on his lips and I love it.

"Beg," Grant growls.

"What? Oh, I mean. Um. I don't understand, Sir," I answer.

"Beg me to give you what you want. What is it you want, pet?"

"I want you to fuck my pussy, Sir. Please, please make me cum."

"You have been a very good girl all night and my cock is throbbing, so I think I'll give you the pleasure of giving me some release." Grant sits up and kneels between my quivering legs. He unbuttons his trousers and slides them off. This is the first time I see his cock. It's a good eight inches and is nice and thick. I don't think I've ever taken a cock this large before and I am slightly nervous, but I am so turned on that I just want to be fucked.

Grant puts the head of his cock in my pussy and I can already feel his size stretching me. In one swift stroke he delves into my pussy to the hilt. I cry out. Not in pain, but in ecstasy. He pounds his hard cock into me. He varies his rhythm and is hitting all the right spots. I can feel my orgasm building. Thankfully, he is moaning louder too.

"Do you want to come, Olivia?" Grant hisses into my ear as he grabs a handful of my hair.

"Yes Sir. Please, make me come." I beg. Grant picks up his pace. I raise my hips to meet his strokes. I am so close.

"Come now!" Grant breathlessly commands. My body explodes into a feeling of pure pleasure. I have never had an orgasm so intense. I am screaming in pleasure.

As I am coming down from my high I feel Grant's body tense and feel him come inside me. He gives out a gruff grunt of pleasure and then collapses on top of me. He rests his head on my breasts while we both catch our breath and regain our composure. He rolls off of me and lays next to me.

After a couple of minutes he gets up and unties my wrists. He pulls me off of the bed, pulls back the covers and then lays me back in the bed. He crawls in next to me and wraps his arms around me. I am in heaven.

He speaks first. "Olivia, that was amazing. I don't know if I'm ever going to let you go." He says with humorous tone. "You can speak freely now."

"I don't think I'll ever want to leave." I say with a smile. "You've given me something that I think I've been searching for my whole life."

PLAYMATES

Frederica Janie de la Fontain

Frederica De La Fontain is a professional massage therapist, amateur photographer and music nerd. When not visiting Disney World she can be found gaming, cooking or begging her husband for sex.

I had turned eight years old during a move across the country with my family. My military father was being transferred from the shipyards of eastern Virginia to the rolling hills of northern California. We were moving away from family and friends to start a new life on a military base outside of San Francisco. Boxes were unpacked and at my mother's urging, my brother and I left the safety of our apartment to seek new friends. Mom had said that the family in the next building over had a girl around my age that I should seek out as a playmate.

Maggie was a few months younger than me, a grade behind me and had a great room full of toys and books. One book she was very proud to show me was called *Where Did I Come From?* which was an explanation about reproduction told in cartoon-style sketches and an easy language for kids to understand. I had never seen anything like this book and was immediately intrigued. My mom had never really explained sex to me but I got the general gist: a man and a woman were needed and it had something to do with the inherent differences in our lower bodies. Until I read that book I didn't even know the proper names for the sexual organs. Growing up in the South, one was taught that those words aren't uttered in polite society. "Tallywhacker," "hoohoo" and "bottom" were the preferred nomenclature. My grandmother said "teetee" instead of "peepee," presumably because the 'p' word meant "piss" where the 't' word stood for "tinkle," which was far more polite.

As my head tried to get around these foreign concepts, I noticed feeling strange sensations when I read the book and looked at the pictures.

Once, we played house and I was the mom and was pretending to put Maggie to bed and she asked to be read The Book. As I read it, I couldn't help but notice that her hands were moving under the blanket, around the area where her crotch was. I didn't say anything but my cheeks flushed red and knew that The Book made her feel funny too, but she didn't care. I don't remember how we got into the conversation, but eventually she turned me on to rubbing myself against things, sliding down the stair railing, spinning around the jungle gym poles with my legs wrapped tightly around it. During a sleepover she was even so bold as to grind against a Coke bottle as it lay on the floor.

Eventually the indirect stimulation was overpowering and we put our hands down our pants, rubbed fast and hard, held our breath, legs straight out, toes pointed and PUSHED...and the tingles just washed over us, like when a car goes over a hill really fast and your stomach does a flip-flop. We would lay on my pink shag rug, panting, fanning ourselves with Rick Springfield album covers, until we caught our breath. Then we would do it again and again, taking turns, until it felt like my heart was going to beat right out of my chest from the exertion.

I found my father's Playboys and Penthouse magazines while looking for socks to borrow. We got a new set of encyclopedias that had clear plastic page overlays of the human anatomical systems. In fifth grade, we were shown movies in school about what happens during puberty and what your period was. We would watch love scenes in movies like *Endless Love* and *The Blue Lagoon* and we would talk about them during sleepovers, eventually acting them out with each other. I even picked her up and carried her, just like a boy did to his girlfriend in *Up the Academy*. We never told anyone, although I think my mom had her suspicions when I would come down to dinner, red-faced and sweating after being in my room for hours.

After a few years, her dad got reassigned to the city and we saw each other infrequently, then my dad got reassigned to Texas. We rented an aging ranch-style house that was plopped in the middle of an upper-class neighborhood. My brother and I knew that we were out of our element compared to these wealthy kids but we tried to play it off. The whole family was experiencing culture shock and at age eleven, I was losing the fight to stay a tomboy. I made friends with some girls that I would be attending school with that Fall and did my best not to make waves. I enrolled in the same dance school as the other girls and tried to assimilate into their idea of style, even though I was clueless. I lived less than an hour from the Pacific Ocean and had no idea what OP or Lightning Bolt clothing was.

There was *one* thing I knew about, that maybe they didn't. One of the girls, Dena, invited me for a sleep over and then her plans changed. Her mom said I could still come over and hang out with her younger sister Katie.

I don't remember how we got on the subject, but there we were, on the foldout sofa bed and I was teaching her what had been taught to me, rubbing, grinding, breathing. She seemed a bit quiet, but I just figured she was shy and didn't know what to do. The next Monday at school, I approached Dena's circle of friends and they turned their backs to me and never spoke directly to me again. I immediately knew why. My mom never said anything to me, so I assume nothing was ever said to her, the matter and I were just...dropped. I got a deep sense of shame about what had happened and

I wondered if Maggie had also looked for another 'playmate' and had gotten busted for it. I never told anyone about this until I was in my twenties, when a friend was looking for validation for her own childhood experiments.

I lost my virginity at age fifteen but I didn't let anyone watch me orgasm again until I was nineteen and I eventually married him. I wasn't going to share that with anyone else that I felt couldn't handle it! I have been in a lot of different sexual relationships, was a swinger with a former boyfriend and experimented with various forms of B/D. I have never had the desire to be with a woman. That experience is part of me, but it doesn't define me. It just was what it was.

SEX AS A FANCY TOOL

Melinda

*I'm a twenty-something, working-class wage slave who
pulls overnight shifts so I can be a stay at home mom
during the day. Married for four years to a wonderful
man who's just as fucked up as I am, only about
different things. Mother to one who had the tenacity to
make it and three that didn't.*

My early life was one long lesson in not trusting
men. I'm the daughter of a single mother who quit
dating once she found out I was on the way. I sat
through the beatings from my grandfather and
watched him do the same to my cousins. Watched
as my uncles beat my aunts and cousins. Watched
as my friends' dads beat them. I was molested in
day care for a year. I used to spend the night at my
best friend's house solely because her dad didn't

have the guts to molest her or her sisters as long as I was there. That same friend and I later narrowly escaped an attempt at gang rape and murder. And the only reason I, unlike many of my friends, didn't barter my body to the neighborhood pedophile was because I knew I'd never be able to come up with a good lie to tell my mom about where I got the Nintendo he was going to give me for services rendered.

All that was before my tenth birthday. When I hit puberty shortly thereafter, I was appalled at the strange new feelings. I wanted to be around boys but I was scared shitless of them. I joined a fundamentalist Christian church because they taught that being gay was a choice. I thought maybe I could take their 'gay cure', reverse it, and live happily as a lesbian. Which of course didn't work. Nine years of trying desperately to be attracted to women only gave me a deep appreciation for breasts. And even then I usually like my own better. I realized that unless I wanted to be alone for the rest of my life, something had to change. Therapy, and lots of it, helped me get over my intense fear of men. One of my assignments from my therapist was to try to make male friends. That was how I met my husband four years ago. We've only ever been with each other, and we've had lots of sex. We were, respectively, twenty-two-and twenty-three-year-old-virgins. We had a lot of catching up to do!

But I have to say that I still don't really 'get' sex. Sure, I enjoy it once we're doing it. I even have great orgasms. But it's always a means to an end for me. I'm emotionally detached from the entire experience, and more than once I've caught myself dissociating mid-coitus. I've never wanted just to have sex. If we're having sex, I have an ulterior motive. That might be trying to conceive. It might be a bribe or hubby's reward for a job well done. Hell, it might even be just to get him to stop whining about why we haven't had sex in a while. I'm ashamed to admit this. I really, really wish I could just get over it already. But I have no idea where to begin, especially since asking for help would mean admitting to my husband that I've never been into it. I want to want it. I just can't seem to figure out how.

P.S.

It's been a year since I originally wrote the above, and I'm a bit ashamed to admit that nothing has changed. It doesn't help that battling infertility made me think of sex as even more of a chore than ever. The years of trying to conceive drilled into me a must-get-pregnant mindset. Two years after finally getting a sticky pregnancy, I still find myself absentmindedly noting the state of my cervical mucus. Still checking out sales on Robitussin, prenatal vitamins, Vitex, and ovulation and pregnancy tests. Still noting every tiny twinge and every spot of blood, and wondering if it's implantation.

But after three miscarriages, life-threatening pregnancy complications with the one that did stick, four days of hellish induced labor, both of us nearly dying during the c-section, then the NICU stay...I cannot do pregnancy again. Not ever. This second-rate baby factory is closed! But because in my fucked-up head, sex = TTC (trying to conceive), I'm scared of it for a whole new reason. And at any rate, having a co-sleeping toddler isn't exactly conducive to working on your sex life. I am still holding out hope that sometime in the future, I'll get the chance to work out my issues. I think I owe it to myself to see how awesome sex can be when you truly want it.

FEMINIST AND SUBMISSIVE?

Picky Britches

Mom. Feminist. Submissive.

I'm a free-thinking, strong-willed, bra-burning feminist. And I'm a bottom in the bedroom. I like to be owned. Stand me in the corner and scold me, please. Excuse me? I know. I get it! How am I furthering the cause for women when I'm bending over and asking to be whipped by a man? Well, here's the thing. I *top* from the bottom. Aren't I clever? You see, being sexually submissive is a choice. It takes great sense of self, enormous trust in my partners, and massive amounts of communication. It is something I want, so I go forth in getting it in a safe manner.

I want to dig a little deeper, and touch on something that I know many people worry about, because I've worried about it myself. Where is the line between being a sub and being a doormat? My partner leaves welts on my ass with his belt, bruises on my thighs where his fingers hold me still. Is this abuse? Not to me. And I know that because I was formerly abused. I was bullied, belittled and raped. Not my choice. Not my fault.

I have found, in my current, safe relationship, that our sexual play has been just the therapy I needed to find myself, to regain my power, and to actually *enjoy* sex again. Logic may say to regain control, it would be therapeutic for me to top a man, to take him in the ass with a strap-on, smack him around, make him my bitch. And yes, for some, that is something they can do in the bedroom, **or dungeon**, that heals them. But for me, with a naturally submissive nature, topping just doesn't feel good.

Just because I'm a rape survivor, just because I was degraded by a former partner, these things do not get to move me out of my natural inclination to be submissive. Being submissive didn't cause those things to happen. They happened because I gave my power to the wrong person and it was abused.

Nothing centers me or brings me more sexual pleasure, than placing myself in my husband's strong hands. We have clear parameters. We communicate constantly. He knows my triggers, and is keenly aware of even the smallest display of body language that says 'danger'. We have a safe word. We discuss our play before it happens. My safety is always at the center.

Being lovingly stroked and cuddled doesn't bring me sexual pleasure. I require intense stimulation and often pain in order to orgasm completely. I love being told what to do and letting go of all my worries and mental lists. I love the headspace where I leave the stress behind and am calmed by being controlled by someone who loves me. Is there something wrong with me? Has abuse molded me into some sort of Stockholm syndrome victim? I used to think so. I used to be so ashamed of what brings me pleasure. Luckily, I've fought through the self-loathing. Life is too short to chastise ourselves, to feel guilty over pleasure. I am who I am: a strong woman, finding pleasure and power from the bottom.

WAKING UP

Nina Potts

Nina Potts is writer from Phoenix, Arizona. She lives there with her partner Dianne and their fur children. She writes stories of her childhood, travels, horror, and erotica. This is her first formally published work. You can learn more about Nina at NinaPotts.com.

I had stopped drinking beer for breakfast. I was still hurting myself, still cutting my arms with my shaving razor once a week. The Ikea bed in our basement suite apartment was always cold, metaphorically and literally. I had become used to the cold, it is one of those things Canada is known for. I had adapted to the weather, though I missed home. I never thought I could miss an Arizona summer. Suddenly I was craving blazing heat on my skin, reminding me of easier times, of an easier life. I wanted to lay on a hot concrete patio as my skin turned pink, to feel the sweat in the small of my back and along my hairline. I wanted that relief of walking into a building and feeling the air conditioner roaring in my face. I really just wanted to feel something other than misery.

Sitting at my work cubicle, feeling exhausted and still slightly drunk from the night before, the headset I was wearing was crackling. I began the irritating task of following cables to electronic bits, trying to find something that would make the headset normal again. Finding nothing, I ducked under my desk. The satin lining of my wool skirt was cool, and barely covered my knees of the scratchy flat carpet. I fiddled with wires and tried to be quiet, even possibly coordinated enough not to bang my head on my desk as I finally reset the power to my computer and phone. It didn't occur to me that I might look strange, on all fours under my desk. As I backed out and pulled myself up, I noticed I was being watched by someone. She looked ridiculous: an orange baseball cap, a lumpy knit sweater with various shades of orange, green and brown striping vertically. Her nose was big, with a slight crook, big lips too. She was staring at me, blatantly, even smiling. It wasn't a friendly smile, more an expression that did not mask what she thought of me in that position. I enjoyed it. It wasn't that I shouldn't enjoy it, it was that I didn't think I could. I felt too dead inside, too constricted trying to hold all of my emotions in check to be presentable to the world.

Months before that day, I discovered that my long-time girlfriend had been cheating on me. I knew. I had known but pushed it away, wanting to ignore it, wanting to take her for her word that she would never. She loved me more because I wasn't her type, even when she cheated on me with girls who were 'her type.' I wanted to be the strong woman who left. I deceived myself, lying to the world that we would work it out. That it was a mistake. I was so caught up in believing the lies I had been fed, that even with proof otherwise I wouldn't give up the perfect life I had created in my mind.

Gita was a rock. No matter how much I tried to lie,

Glitter

she broke in. Just that look on her face, staring at me in some smug, amused, slightly sexual way, put the first small crack in my mental image of my life. I didn't like her. She was rude, brash, and loud. When she walked she stomped, big combat boots or tennis shoes, I could hear her coming down the hallway at work. She was short, too short. And bald. And she smoked. And she stared at me every day like she was having sex with me while I was working. I talked to her at work, and even gave her my phone number. She wanted to have sex with me, and let me know it. I liked it, feeling desired, feeling like I was someone worthy of having. She wanted to take me out for coffee, and didn't care that I had a girlfriend.

I said yes to coffee. I told her up front that I was not going to have sex with her. I wasn't interested. It was just coffee, and a walk to the beach. In my head I reminded myself that I wasn't sleeping with her. She wasn't attractive enough, but there was something. Her swagger, the way she guided me with her hand at my lower back when we walked downhill. She walked on the street side, old fashioned chivalry with a booming laugh. She held nothing back, and did not care what anyone thought, letting every thought out. I liked the flirting and the attention more and more. I liked the look on her face when I told her I was kinky, that I wrote erotica, and I wanted to be spanked. We were at the beach so long. It got dark, and even colder. I let her kiss me, and that submissive part of me began waking up, sinking down to let her take over. I let her take me into her small apartment, I let her spank me.

Every moment after that blurs into days and weeks of tawdry, passionate, kinky sex that trashy romance novels are made of. I didn't run away from my girlfriend to her, and she didn't ask me to. I didn't hide what I was doing either. I practically paraded her in front of my girlfriend, as proof that I was good enough for someone. A part of me felt justified. The rest was a chaos of resolution, disgust at my weakness in staying with someone who lied so much, self-awareness, and the sexual gratification I had craved all along but never finding someone who could be what I needed.

I remember the exact moment I decided I couldn't stay with Terri anymore. I was riding the bus home from work, looking at the buildings and shops. Crowds of people together. I felt so calm. I knew that I couldn't stay with Terri anymore. I also knew it was time to go home.

I moved out of our apartment, I took my dog, and accepted Gita's offer to stay with her for the month until I moved back to Arizona. That single month was the best time I lived in Vancouver. I became attracted to those things about her before that turned me off. I liked her baldness, and the way she stomped when she walked. I liked that she was ten years older than me. She was Lebanese, and I liked hearing her slight accent suddenly start when she talked to her mother on the phone. She quit smoking even before our first date because I didn't like it, and I didn't know. I loved how butch she was, and that she was proud of it too. I loved her rough hands. I didn't want gentleness, secrets, or lies. There was no way to lie to her, she saw through it, she saw when I was lying to myself. Mostly, she saw me in a sexual way. I spent that month talking, eating, and shedding years of repressed sexual energy.

Gita and I had both been involved in BDSM before, but never in a relationship, and our conversations were completely honest. Neither of us were formally trained, which did cause some issues. We didn't know about aftercare, but our scenes always led to sex which led to resting together after, so in our own way we did have aftercare. We found our way. My every fantasy was open to her. We flowed in and out of our Daddy/girl roles when together, whether in the bedroom, out walking, or having dinner. Everything felt natural and easy, calming part of the chaos I was trying to tame.

We role played my ultimate fantasy at the time, which involved myself as a teenage girl, with a teacher who convinced me to give him my virginity. Just acting it out I could barely follow the scene. I wanted so much to be touched and taken right away. She kept me in my place until exactly when she wanted me, stripping me down, taking advantage of me and responding just as I had played the scene in my mind a million times.

When slightly alone she could hardly keep her hands off me. I have an exhibitionist streak, and working in the same office made that dangerous. I loved sneaking to the bathroom, her hand over my mouth to keep me quiet, with our boss in the next stall over. I wore skirts more often. I laid on her couch reading Shakespeare naked, teasing her when she was busy with paperwork and bills.

She quickly learned that I had multiple girl sides, one a non-sexual little girl who loved to play and color, and another, bratty sexual teenager. We both found out that I would misbehave to be punished, which made her stop punishing me. I soon wanted to do nothing more than make her happy all the time, and leaving Vancouver became harder.

I had wanted to have a fun fling and go home to heal. I didn't expect to develop feelings that might even be love. I didn't think I could love someone so quickly, when I was still so broken inside. I extended my stay a few more weeks, saying that I wasn't ready to see my family after a failed relationship. I surprised her with a tiny Charlie-Brown-type Christmas tree. We got each other gifts, a watch for her that I knew she would love, and a digital camera for me. It wasn't what I had originally wanted, but it was brilliant. I had so many pictures to take home with me, of her, my friends, and all of my favorite places in Vancouver. When I got home I could send her pictures of

Arizona, my friends, and teasing pictures of myself in various outfits or positions. She wanted me to come back, to get married so I could stay. We had an argument that night. We both had quick and loud tempers, and her studio apartment filled with shouts about my changing my name if we got married. It was a part of me I couldn't give up, I couldn't change my name. It was me, it was where I came from, I couldn't give that away. We made up, but it stayed with me, a worry in the back of my mind.

After New Year's I came back to Arizona. It was harder than I thought to leave. Part of me wanted to stay, but the parts that were still broken were calling me home.

I stayed with my best friend until I found a job and apartment. Gita and I had decided to have an open relationship. Neither of us were jealous sorts of people, and we both understood that having sex with someone else did not have to have a relationship attached to it. I had fun, my best friend was single, I liked going out and hitting on girls with her. Gita liked hearing of my exploits, the dirty things I let others do to me. No matter how anyone touched me, I was still her girl, and she was still my Daddy.

We were so drawn to each other, and the sexual attraction so deep that I was only home three weeks before she surprised me with a plane ticket to visit her. I went back to Vancouver for two weeks. We both had bought some books on BDSM and were eager to use our new expertise.

She was still working early mornings when we rented movies one night. For my teenage girl side she got *The Princess Diaries* 2. She needed a nap, and had no desire to watch the movie. I couldn't help giggling during the movie, unintentionally waking her. She instructed me to be quiet, or she would duct tape my mouth, which she knew I didn't like the smell of the tape. I was so good, so quiet. When the movie was over I carefully and silently went to turn it off. She woke up, and before I could think about it a hushed "hi" slipped out. I knew I was in trouble, even if it was an accident, my eyes wide I clamped my hand over my mouth. I don't remember what her movie was that we stayed up to watch, but I remember the smell of the tape on my mouth. I stayed quiet and still, trying not to fidget. Afterward she rewarded me, taking me from behind with her strap-on, letting me be as loud as I wanted.

We pretended to be tourists on her day off before I left, visiting Granville Island, and the Aquarium at Stanley Park. We made plans for me to return in a few months with some saved-up money, get married and work on changing my citizenship. We didn't talk about the name change issue. The day I left again, I was supposed to take the bus to the airport. She surprised me again, calling a taxi and riding with me, savoring every last moment we had.

I came home and started a job with an airline in their call center. I made more friends, including another Daddy/girl couple. Being around them made me feel safe and sane, when I knew so few people could understand Gita and I. There was still all of my baggage from my past relationship that surfaced every day. Somehow, in trying to put myself back together, to see if those pieces of me that broke were still me, I got lost. I had old feelings for my best friend, and I knew she had them for me. If I had been honest with myself, paid attention to how I felt inside, I would have known that it was a mistake. Gita was furious, but I dated my best friend anyways.

She called me a liar, and I was. I didn't know it, that I was lying to myself, and I had lied to her. I thought those feelings for my best friend were gone, when our relationship at college ended, it still left untied strings. I thought we could put them back together, even though I knew that she wasn't into BDSM and couldn't be that for me. She wanted to be that, but it wasn't in her. I ruined our friendship, breaking up with her only a few weeks later, feeling horrible about myself. I felt like I had taken advantage of the feelings she had for me, and my need to be with someone who wanted me that was not a whole country away.

I spent over a year trying to figure out what I needed. I made a mental checklist of things I wanted in a person. I learned how to take care of myself before anyone else. I lost my way a few more times. I had one night stands. While with Terri I had been a stripper for some time, financially supporting us. I went back to it, and although I was in a better mindset this time, it made me colder inside. Having to separate myself from who I was and who I needed to be at work. I found a new best friend, another femme. I had friends that were close, that I could confide in. That person that I was still becoming when I met Terri, and lost while trying to be what she wanted, suddenly was here. I was me, I knew what I liked and didn't like. I knew when I did something why I was doing it, and to self-reflect. The little girl part of me was lonely, and the adult part of me felt like I needed to talk to Gita again.

After a few phone calls we picked up where we left off. It was like we had never been separated. True to her nature, she surprised me again and came to visit just after Christmas. I loved showing her where I came from, the things I loved about Arizona. I loved waking up feeling safe and protected every day. She loved my new best friend, and being out with us made Gita feel proud with two sexy femmes by her side. I wasn't broken inside anymore, I was stronger.

I had started missing Vancouver since I left, feeling like I had two homes. I wanted to split myself so I could live in both. With Gita back in my life there was the pressure to move back to Vancouver. I told her I didn't want to get married, that it was something I wasn't sure I ever wanted to do. It was too dangerous to do just for me to get citizenship. I couldn't guarantee to her or myself that things would work out between us enough to take that risk.

I visited again, for only a week that time. Going back to Vancouver was amazing, but this was Gita's home. I had been through so many things while we were apart, while she visited Arizona it was like a fun vacation. Now that I was where she lived, I saw the cracks again in our relationship. I saw this strange possessiveness that hadn't been there before. I discovered she had been using drugs, and lied about some of the things she did when I was gone. My sexual and BDSM experience had increased ten-fold, and I couldn't fit her into what I wanted in a Daddy anymore. I came back to Arizona conflicted and disenchanted. I thought I had become the person I needed to be when we were together before. Perhaps I was, but she wasn't what I needed anymore. I felt less attracted. She felt me pulling away, even over the phone. It may be why she became so possessive, calling me constantly, checking up on me, desperately grasping for me as I drifted away.

I had fallen asleep on my couch one night, sick, exhausted from work. My cell phone was next to me, but I had it on silent. She called me fifty-one times that night. The voice mails ranged from worried to outraged. I was frightened, and suddenly grateful that she was so far away. The next day, on the phone was just yelling, insulting me, trying to tear me down, that I was a liar, and a gold digging whore. I was already gone. I had nothing to say. I couldn't be her girl when as a Daddy and a girlfriend she was losing control.

It's been seven years since then. I don't think of her often, but I remember the good times the most. That first spanking, walking on her arm in downtown Vancouver on our way to dinner, the intense late-night conversations, and the first time I blushingly called her Daddy.

It's Just Sex

Bella

Single mother, variety performer, and theatrical producer who came of age in the 90's.

The night I was supposed to be finishing up my Glitter submission, I was having booty call sex with a dwarf instead. Ten years ago I would have considered that sentence a punchline. Now it's my life.

The first part of my childhood was spent being raised by my Mexican Catholic grandparents. It was a very loving, but horribly repressed environment. When I was eight I moved in with my 29-year-old father and spent the rest of elementary school and all of high school under his incredibly strict, emotionally unavailable tutelage. My mother had been MIA since I was three, thanks to the fact that she enjoyed locking me in a closet while she got high with her gentleman caller of choice for that week. My stepmother was kind at times, but seemed to mostly view me as a source of resentment. Any psychological study will tell you it's no surprise that I went into show business. Or that I enjoy rough sex and bondage.

Trust me, I tried to conform. I tried to be the good little Catholic girl who was also devoted to her family. I became a wife at 21. The moment it came to walk down the aisle I knew it wasn't what I wanted to do, but I felt it was too late. Too much money. Too many guests. Too much riding on that day and my shoulders to make my family proud. Besides, the church was beautiful and I looked great in my dress, so I went through with it and stayed in it for eight incredibly unhappy and unfulfilled years. I was miserable, a shell of a human being, and a huge bitch. I would say I lost eight years of my life, but to be honest, those years shaped everything that my life is now. There are two reasons I can never call my marriage a mistake. The first reason is my daughter who was born when I was 26. She is an amazing child. Her spirit is gorgeous and she is everything a person should be. The tears stinging my eyes as I type are a testament to the pure, unconditional love I have for this little girl. Being her mother has taught me what connection and family really is and I will forever be grateful to her for that.

The second reason is what this story is really about. Me. After I separated from my ex-husband, I began to really discover who I was. I don't think that would have happened had I not been so unhappy to begin with. My divorce began the realization of what my life truly was meant to be. I discovered theatre again and then slowly began to discover vaudeville, variety, sideshow, and circus. I finally figured out how to release all the art that had always been inside me. Sharing my theatrical visions, my body, my voice, and my soul keeps my heart alive. One of the effects of feeling so great and being so comfortable in my own skin? Great sex. Once I started to love every part of myself, inside and out, my sexual encounters became more fulfilling than ever before.

I lost my virginity at 17 on the floor of my bedroom one weekday afternoon. From that two minute experience on, every intimate moment was about trying to get the love and attention that my father had never bestowed on me. So, in essence, I was having sex for my dad. In case you didn't know, having that idea in the back of your head really hinders trying to get off. Learning to love myself and coming to terms with the lack of relationship between my father and I gave me the freedom to focus on pleasure. Up until I was 32, I had never had sex outside of a committed relationship. One night stands were not in my database. Again, it was because sex wasn't about pleasure for me. It was about fierce attempts to gain intimacy and acceptance. Losing that crutch opened me up to realize that sex can be JUST SEX. That was amazing. The booty call mentality is so liberating. I'm still picky about who I choose to engage with. I love pleasure and excitement, but I love my health more. Plus the fact that I have plenty to live for and a little girl who counts on me is more than enough to ensure that I'm always careful.

A dear male friend of mine put it best when I expressed the fact that I was surprised about how comfortable I had become with sex and multiple partners. He said, 'You're doing what most people do in their twenties, except you're in your thirties and being smart about it. That's good.' He's right. I see my sexual liberation as empowering. That sentence feels so cliche, but it's true. Knowing that my body is beautiful and that it deserves to be ravished and worshiped makes finding pleasure easy and fun. Bondage used to be a way to escape responsibility. If I was helpless during sex, it removed all traces of Catholic guilt. Now I relish the fact that I love the way leather straps feel against my skin. The sting of a whip followed by the caress of a gentle hand is heavenly.

I no longer have shame in admitting my fetishes. I have no shame in admitting I love sex. I love the exploration and the excitement of the new. This is not to say that I will never again enter into a committed relationship. Some day, I know I'll find the right person to grow old with. The best part is knowing that when I do find that person, our sex life is going to rock. He will learn what my body responds to and enjoys because I won't be afraid to ask for it. It will be a life of acceptance and love because I accept and love myself. I am a confident and powerful woman who isn't afraid to take risks or to push the social taboos of a repressed society. And thank god for that, because my dwarf is one of the best lovers I've ever had.

FIRSTS

Lauren Marie Fleming

Lauren Marie Fleming (aka Queerie Bradshaw) writes about sex, politics, the law, and sometimes shoes, at QueerieBradshaw.com. Her writing has also been featured in CurveMag.com, Autostraddle.com, Vice.com and Nerve.com. This is an excerpt from her upcoming autobiography.

> *The first kiss is where you get to know someone. And every kiss after that is a shadow of that first one.*

Betty Draper (January Jones), *Mad Men*

My very first kiss was in preschool for a popsicle. I don't remember the kiss much, but I do remember that popsicle. Then there was the plethora of spin the bottle type games, including a special one we made up called 'pass the tic-tac', my personal favorite. The first real one happened when I was twelve. He touched my boobs, I touched his thingy, it was hormonal and full of the insecurities of puberty. When I kissed my first woman a few years later, I was even more nervous and excited than I had been at twelve.

One would think that this awkwardness would go away, but it hasn't. Reaching that first kiss with someone is still just as thrilling for me as it had been back in junior high. The slow movement forward, checking to see if they want it as much as you do, praying they want it as much as you do, then the excitement as you feel that they do want it as much as you do. Kissing used to be such an intimate thing for me that I would save it only for very special people. Periods of my life have been marked by anti-kissing decrees and I have had sex with people without our lips ever touching.

Nowadays, I'm not as anti-intimacy as I used to be, but I'm still just as sensitive to kissing. I can tell how much I like a girl by how long it takes me to kiss her. If she makes my clit throb, I'll grab her and have at it right then and there. But if she makes my heart twitter, I may never even attempt a hug. The night I first kissed Tsunami, we laid in bed, slowly getting closer and closer, until we finally had no choice but to meet. The tension was so strong I thought nothing could ever top it.

Then I kissed The Wind.

Over a year of flirtatious texting and intimate conversations led us to finally meet in her bed late one cold San Francisco evening. Cuddled up in every blanket she owned, I spent hours naming her body parts in Italian until she finally let my lingua meet hers. The Wind had a way of making each kiss feel like a first. The tease and tension of her tongue kept me in anticipation for years, and the dark shadow kisses Betty Draper talks of never crept their way into our love life. The mouths that I've met since The Wind have been nice, but nothing has blown my socks off in the stomach churning intestinal twisting way hers used to.

It was thinking about that kiss that made me start missing The Wind. But more than that, it made me start missing intimacy and physicality with an emotional connection. Masturbating is great, it really is, but there is no machine to replace kissing, trust me, I've looked. So, I upped my game, looking to find someone to kiss.

I like to think that I am smooth at picking up a gal, but I'm really not. It's so hard to go up to someone and ask for their phone number. I've gotten better at it for sure, but at this point in my story I was still batting zero for taking home a girl from a bar. The cheesy pick-up lines never work on me, so I assume they don't work on others either. Sure, my dad may have stolen the stars and put them in my eyes, I may have lost that loving feeling and I'm sorry you've lost your number, but you are going to have to come up with a line less canned and more honest if you want to take me home. And I knew I was going to have to come up with something unique for other girls as well.

Thinking it might be my in, the angle that wins me the gals, I tried the whole "I'm a sex blogger, I'd love to write about you" thing online to a few people I thought were hot. I can't blame them for never emailing me back. When that failed, I tried it on a waif blonde in a leather jacket and dark makeup at a local lesbian bar. The minute I saw her walk in, I was smitten and talking to her took mustering up all the courage I had in my body. In the most nonchalant, confident manner I could handle, I did this:

Me: "You're gorgeous. What's your name?"

Her: "_____" (This isn't blank for anonymity. Being horrible with names, I have actually blanked on what hers was.)

Me: "Hello, _____, I'm Queerie Bradshaw. Are you single?"

Her: "Yes, I'm single."

Me: "Would you like to go out on a date sometime?"

Her: "It's new." (Meaning she's newly single, I rightfully assumed.)

Me: "That's cool. Want to hang out as friends sometime instead?"

Her: "Sure. I guess that would be fine."

Me: "Would it be pretentious if I gave you my card?"

Her: "No."

Me: "Here's my card. I'm Queerie."

Her: "I got that the first time. I gotta go see my friends. Bye."

That is literally the whole interaction we had at the bar. I, not too shockingly, never heard back from her. I have a long way to go before I'm Rico Suave with the ladies. I was short and nervous, and should have asked for her number instead of giving her mine. Rookie mistakes. At least I tried with her, though. The day before this, I went to a Mexican food restaurant and spent the whole time drooling over the tatted up butch behind the counter. I talked to her, flirted a bit, and then left without saying a word about my desire to have her take tequila shots off of my naked body. I've always been told it's impolite to hit on people while they're working, especially if they're serving you, but as soon as I left I regretted my manners.

I'm beginning to think it takes a bit of some pushy brusqueness to pick up a stranger. Maybe that's just what years of watching romantic comedies has taught me, but maybe there actually is something to the bold, outlandish pick-ups I've heard about. My new theory is that blatantly hitting on people is more successful than subtle seduction. I'm starting to believe that Joey Tribbiani on Friends had it right when he'd sit down uninvited next to a girl at a bar, give her a smirk and say "How you doin'?"

Forward, blunt, sassy and honest may be the best way to go, and the best place to go for that is the internet.

Tired of striking out at bars and coming home with only boxes of toys and my thoughts for company, I put two ads on Craigslist at the same time: one searching for "Just Friends" and the other searching for "Just Sex." Ironically, the responses to the Just Friends ad produced creepiness ("I've lived here for six years, it would be nice to finally have a friend") and the Just Sex ad introduced me to some fun new people.

When up in Portland for burlesque gigs or a simple escape from Eugene, I often studied – yes, I actually studied during this whorish period of mine – at a cute little patisserie on Alberta street named Le Petite Provence. The waiters knew me and we chatted often about legal ethics and croissant ingredients. I was safe and in my element there and so I asked Costello, the most promising responder to my "Just Sex" ad to meet me there. Costello's response to my ad was sexual without being creepy, and after a few interactions on email, I knew I liked her; which was why I was shockingly nervous as I sat there waiting for her to show up for a quick tea date.

I know that I'm a big bad sex and dating blogger and I should be able to go out into cafés around the world with confidence and ladies on my arms, but the reality is dating is a scary thing. As I waited for

Costello to show up, the story of the Stone Butch Daddy (SBD), one of my very first, first dates, went reeling through my mind.

It wasn't exactly a blind date, but it may as well have been. I was working the door at Miss Kitty's Scratching Post, a monthly lesbian strip club in San Francisco, when we met. I wore a camo corset, lacy bottoms, fishnets, platform shoes and a sticker that said "Ask Me for My Number." That outfit got me two dates, one with the fabulous performer Alotta Boutté (who later became one of my best friends) and the other with SBD (who I avoid to this day).

On her way out of the club, SBD approached me and asked if I liked ice cream. I replied that I love ice cream. She then asked if I liked motorcycles, and, like the good little SF femme I was, I replied of course. Then SBD asked if I wanted to go get ice cream with her on her Harley.

I creamed my pants and gave her my number.

The day of the date, SBD called me to say that the Harley wasn't available after all. Turns out she didn't actually own a Harley, she just worked in a Harley repair shop and thought she could borrow one for the night. Strike one. Begrudgingly, I agreed to pick her up. If I wasn't getting a Harley, at least I was getting some ice cream. Yet, it turned out ice cream was out of the question too. She was hungry, and insisted we go get some sushi instead. Strike two.

Strike three through ten happened while waiting for an hour and a half outside in the cold SF fog at the particular sushi joint she had to go to, even though the one down the street was great and had no wait. Once inside, she refused to let me order for myself, told me she was my daddy and it was her job to make decisions for me, and that she thought I'd make perfect arm candy to take back to live in the back country of Hawaii while she grew pineapples and I made dinner and watched her work on her (nonexistent) Harley.

At least she paid.

The complete disappointment that came from SBD led to my future fear of first dates. I thought I was getting ice cream on the back of a Harley, but instead got myself into what was a now humorous but then horrible situation. As I sat and waited for Costello to arrive, the 'what if' worm dug its way through my brain thinking of all the ways this date could top that first date in ridiculousness. So what did I do when Costello arrived? I awkwardly spewed the whole story of SBD as soon as she sits down.

I've been told I'm an over-sharer before, giving way too many details than needed and speaking of things most people consider highly private. I've been told this often makes people uncomfortable around me. Luckily for both of us, Costello found the story to be funny. I liked her instantly for this. I liked her instantly for many reasons, most of which centered around her sharp sense of humor.

Once, when I first came out, I posted an ad on Craigslist seeking another female for a date. When I showed up for that date, the person turned out to be a creepy guy impersonating a girl to try to get lesbians to sleep with him. When I turned him down, he told me I was a sinner and he was going to give me his cock to save me from hell, but now that I turned it down I would instead burn. This is just one example of the multitude of experiences I've had with men impersonating women online, this is just a sampling of the kind of shit lesbians put up with regularly.

That guy's cock may not have saved me from eternal damnation like he had planned, but it did save me from many other potentially dangerous dates. He taught me the importance of meeting in familiar public places and having an escape route. My date with Costello was no exception to this rule. I chose Le Petite Provence because the waiters knew me well and I planned a meeting an hour after our rendezvous so I had an excuse to leave if things went badly.

But things did not go badly. They went the opposite of badly. They went swimmingly. We got along so well that I invited Costello to accompany me to a burlesque show that evening. The show must have not been too impressive because I only vaguely remember it. Was I in I or was I just watching? I know Pumpkin was there and that

Costello and Pumpkin got along wonderfully as well, which was a good sign to me. I remember there was a lot of laughing. And maybe we all danced together. I'm not sure about the dancing, but I am sure that I wanted to invite myself over to Costello's house that night. Badly.

The problem with being a law student was everyone started expecting legal help from me. I wasn't allowed to give legal advice until I passed the bar, but that didn't stop people from asking for it. At the very least, I was still on the hook for emotional and intellectual support in the legal realm when friends needed it. A friend of mine and his boyfriend had recently ended their relationship with a fist fight, a call to the cops and restraining orders. The next morning, I was supposed to get up early and accompany him to his hearing. His need for help and my brain's need for sleep before I encountered a judge on the bench trumped my desire to go home with Costello and so I went home alone, without even a kiss.

It was two weeks before I made it back to Portland and by that time Costello and I were ready to go. We had emailed and texted constantly and the sexual tension was good and tight. We met for dinner at a Thai place that had better reviews than the food deserved, and talked for an awkwardly long time after our meals were done. For a reason I can't remember, we decided we just had to go teeter-tottering, and went to a local park to satisfy our craving. I'd hoped for some slide or swing sex, but alas, no moves were made, just awkward moments of tense hesitation.

Still dizzy from spinning swings, we went back to her place under the pretense of seeing what On Demand had in the way of movies. Pretense turned into reality, though, when we made it through the whole fabulously campy *Spice World* without a single wandering hand. Again, just awkward moments of tense hesitation.

Moving on to looking at sex toy websites, I inched closer to her yet still didn't feel a response. When we started looking at porn sites without a move being made, I thought we were doomed.

"Fuuuuuuck," I thought. "Fuuuuuuuck" screamed my vagina. "Fuuuuuuuuuuuuck" screamed pretty much every part of me. "FUCK IT!" screamed my head and finally I just leaned over, a bit too fast and forcefully, and kissed her.

I let out a loud sigh of relief when she kissed me back.

Grabbing and kissing someone is scary. Slowly moving towards each other makes it obvious the other person wants it too so there's less of a chance you'll get rejected, but if you're getting nothing from the body language it's a frightening prospect to boldly go where you haven't gone before. It should have been obvious she wanted me too, we had talked about it for a while and in some detail, yet there was a part of me, the majority part of me, that was still shocked when her lips showed an interest in mine. No matter how many people I sleep with, no matter how many cheers I get as I take my clothes off on a stage, no matter how many people I have in my life that love me, I will always continue to be shocked when someone likes me. As the past fades and I no longer hear my father's voice telling me how unattractive my body is, my mother's voice telling me how unattractively obnoxious and stubborn my personality is, maybe a bit of that shock will fade with it. As I move away from my childhood home of quick-fix dieting and single-minded goals, as I swim farther from the fish bowl and into the sea, maybe I'll begin to see that I am likable, lovable and desirable, even though I was an awkward, fat, loud, nonconforming little girl. Maybe one day I will see that I am likable, lovable and desirable precisely because I am an awkward, fat, loud and nonconforming woman.

But that night, in the room with Costello, I wasn't there yet. Writing this, I am still not there yet and so I am still shocked, as I was then, when someone likes me enough to kiss me.

Costello's kiss did give me enough confidence to garner hope that this would go farther and soon I had blue ovaries to go with that confidence. I thought that once we breached the first kiss we would rip each other's clothes immediately off and go at it like wild rabbits, but again, things moved slowly with awkward moments of tense hesitation. Each step took time and prodding on my part. She wasn't being prudish by any means, but she definitely didn't move as fast as I was used to. I was there with a goal and something was impeding my victory. As each minute passed, fear set in, a fear of having to come back here and do this again, a fear of a continued connection.

I liked Costello. The longer it took me to get what I came there for, the greater the chance that like would turn into something more, something less stable, something less cut and dry. As of now, we were people who met on Craigslist with one goal: fucking. The longer I stayed in bed with Costello, joking, laughing, rolling around and kissing, the higher that chance that other goals would form. And I did not have room in my life for any more goals.

Some say it's good for me to learn to slow down, but my body was not in agreement. My legs had shut down from being open for painfully long, and my mind was starting to join them, leading to boredom and annoyance. The time for pussy footing was over. Now was the time for pussy pounding. Using every part of my body, including my voice, I expressed to Costello that I wanted her inside of me. Now. I didn't care which cock she used, I didn't care which condom she put on it, I didn't care how her harness was attached, I just wanted her in me that very second.

I let out a neighbor-waking moan when I finally felt her slip inside.

Thrust, thrust, thrust, moan, moan, moan, glory, glory, glory hallelujah it was finally happening. My goal was finally met. Whatever happened from this point on didn't matter. We could take as long as Costello wanted now that I had what I wanted. My belt was notched, my box was checked, now I could get on with enjoying the ride.

Except, I couldn't really enjoy the ride, not with my legs so sore and stiff from the hours of dry humping we already did on Costello's couch. I'm quite flexible and usually great at opening my legs for someone, but tonight my body had given up. As Costello thrust on top of me, I groaned both in pleasure and in pain. I had finally gotten what I wanted and I couldn't enjoy it. I hopped on top, thinking that controlling the movement between my thighs might help stop the burning in them, but soon my hips were complaining too. Just when I thought I was going to have to give up and stop, Costello said, "I want to use my hand."

Oh thank god, I thought, closing my legs to a more comfortable position. Costello's hands did not require my legs to be wide open. Costello grabbed a latex glove and some lube, then slowly, one finger at a time, entered me again. Strapping it on is fun, it allows the hands to stay free and makes for a closer connection with your partner, but nothing compares to the variety, specification and adaptability of fingers. Fingers can do five things. Fingers can go five ways. Fingers can take me five different places. All at once. And Costello had very talented fingers. Flipping on my back, she worked me so hard her bed rolled its way across her wooden floor to the other side of the room. All my eagerness for hurrying before was drained out of me, I never wanted this to stop. But Costello was now the pushy one, Costello was now speeding, taking me up, up, up, fast, fast, fast. I had no choice but to go along for the ride. Grabbing a pillow, I covered my mouth and screamed as I went over the edge.

We went for more until my legs gave out and we both collapsed exhaustingly onto her bed. We laid for a bit deciding how to feed our growling stomachs (it had been almost twelve hours since that unsatisfying Thai dinner), but exhaustion won over and we soon passed out. I woke up with a start a few minutes later, realizing I was asleep in a practical stranger's bed. Even more startling, however, was the realization that I wanted to stay there, that I wanted to get to know this charming stranger. This was a first for me and like my first kiss and my first date, I felt awkward and scared. There was an opportunity for depth, an opportunity for growth, and I consciously ran away from it, choosing once again persona over personal. Queerie Bradshaw did not spend the night, she came and went. So I got up, got dressed, and got out of there in as polite of a way as possible.

It was six a.m., and both the sun and my friends on the East Coast were up. On my trek across town, I called and regaled a few New Yorkers with tales of the evening and thirty minutes later, exhaustingly dragged my body up the stairs and into bed next to Pumpkin, the only person whose bed I could share. He was just coming home himself and we chatted about our mutual morning ménages before passing out with smiles on our faces and pain in our thighs.

Over the next month or so, I made half-assed attempts to get back up to Portland and see Costello, but between finals and packing for my summer internship in San Francisco, it never really worked out. Eventually, we morphed into friendland and that's where we've been ever since. I can't deny I thought about what it would be like to date her, how it would feel to open up to her, how things might be different if I had stayed in her bed that evening, but there is a time and a place for that emotional depth and I was not ready for anything more that evening in Costello's bed.

THE POWER OF SHAME

Mona Darling

Mona Darling aka Dead Cow Girl, spent close to twenty years as an A-list Professional Dominatrix before becoming a D-list Mommy Blogger. After spending many years traveling the world being told that she is fabulous, she now spends her days being told she doesn't drive fast enough by her three-year-old son.

My uncle just called me a cum bucket on our private family Facebook group. I really don't want to call him 'my' anything and I guess if I were to call him my something, I should call him my childhood bully or even my childhood molester.

And yes. The irony of my childhood molester calling adult me a cum bucket is not lost on me.

I realize when I dismiss it lightly, that people look at me strangely. But he no longer holds any power over me, so him calling me names is really just a waste of time on his part. It doesn't hurt me and it makes him look the fool.

I'm considering this a defining moment in my sexual history NOT because it defined my ideas around sex, but defined my ideas about the shame surrounding sex, because the actual abuse wasn't bad. It was the shame and the guilt that did the damage. I guess that's why I'm a fanatic for removing the shame from both sex and abuse.

Not that I think everyone should run around having sex with everyone else, I feel, quite strongly, that each person's sexual proclivities, habits and desires are to be respected. There is no shame in being monogamous, polyamorous, kinky or vanilla, gay, straight, bi or celibate, slut or virgin, it's your decision, and it's a very personal one.

My uncle was several years older than me and always a bully. Obviously still is. I was five, living with my grandparents while my mom dealt with other things, and I was terrified of him. Some of it was simple boy-teasing-girl things: sticking a frog in my bed while I was sleeping. Threatening to dip my hand in water and make me pee my pants if I went to sleep on the couch. Convincing me that I could ride my trike down a very steep road.

And in fact I was a big ol' cry baby if I didn't do it.

I still have little scars in my knees from when I landed. They have faded with time and only I know they are there at this point, probably more in my mind, than in actual visible proof.

The only time this bully was nice to me was when he and his friends would corner me in some distant part of the yard, behind a shed or bush, and tell me to take my pants down so they could see at my girlie parts. I was terrified of them, but once I did it, my five-year-old brain was thrilled that I had finally found a way to make this bully like me, to make him be nice to me, at least for a moment.

I don't remember how many times it happened. Nor do I remember how far it went. I don't want to. I don't care. I do remember it was a fairly common activity. I remember one time he tried to bully me into getting into sexual positions with the neighbor's dog, but thankfully his friends decided that was going too far. He promised to make me do it later when they weren't around to protect me.

I didn't tell then, because I wanted him to like me.

One time my grandmother came around the corner and caught us. Me with my pants down, him and a friend staring.

Laughing.

She chastized me and demanded I pull my pants up as he explained that I had been following them around doing it all day. Bugging them. That I did it all the time.

I was banished to my room for the rest of afternoon, not to protect me from my uncle, but because my grandmother thought, at five, that I was so promiscuous that I needed protection from myself.

I didn't tell then, because I thought I'd done something wrong.

As time went on and I moved away, back with my mother to another state, I pushed it to the back of my mind, which had twisted it into "that's the uncle I explored with." Even though it was 100% one-sided.

And because it was 100% one-sided, because there was no traditional penis-in-mouth/hand/vagina, I never thought of him as molesting me.

After all, he didn't do anything. I was the one who pulled my pants down. But more than anything, I didn't want anyone to know that I had, at one time, wanted this bully to like me.

I didn't tell then, because I was ashamed of what I had done.

Any time I was around him for family vacations, reunions, and finally, when we moved to the same city, I had a hard time being friendly. I felt I was the butt of all his jokes. I was scared that at some point, in the middle of some self-aggrandizing tirade, that he would tell the family about how I used to pull my pants down to entertain him.

The family thought I was being too sensitive. He was, after all, everyone's favorite uncle. The baby of that generation, doted on by the elders, looked up to by the youngsters.

It was just me that looked at him in terror and distrust.

I didn't tell then, because who would believe me?

After all, it was so long ago.

And after all, it was just kids exploring.

It's natural. Right?

It wasn't until recently almost forty years later, that I realized that what he did was not ok. That it wasn't my fault. That I didn't bring it upon myself.

I wonder if my grandmother knew and just didn't want to deal with it. If it was easier for her to ignore her child being a horrible bully then to address the issue with me. I wonder if she ever thought that she should have handled it another way or if she just pushed it from her mind.

Or maybe that's why she didn't trust me when I was a teenager.

I sometimes wonder what the rest of the family would say. To this day I have not told a soul. You, dear reader, are the first, the only people to know. There is no reason to tell. He would never be punished. I would be further shamed.

I'm not entirely certain how this whole event shaped me. I've spent a lot of time thinking about that over the last couple months as I tried to decide what to write about as MY defining moment. Perhaps this is one reason why I like to be in control sexually. As a switch, I am able to find power in topping or bottoming. Either side is about being desired.

Maybe it's why I found sex work to be an easy and exciting career. I found a way to get people to like me. Even the bullies.

That's a double-edged sword though. Because for everyone who likes me because I'm a sex worker, there is someone I can't tell for fear they will shame me.

I don't want to think that he did anything to shape me, aside from being a perfect bad example of a human being. And I don't want to think that he did anything to shape my sexual desires. I feel those desires are mine and they are very personal. I feel that I have explored the world, my self, my lovers, friends and slaves and I have found what I like and enjoy. I have explored my limits and think I know where and what they are. I have worked hard to find out what turns me on and to get past any shame associated with it.

Maybe I'm lucky to see it that way. Maybe I'm just so messed up that I don't realize what kind of damage he did to me.

Either way, I am me and I am my own imperfect creation.

ABOUT THE EDITOR

Mona Darling spent close to twenty years as an A-list professional dominatrix before becoming a D-list mommy blogger. After spending many years traveling the world being told that she is fabulous, she now spends her days being told she doesn't drive fast enough by her three-year-old son.

She is also a certified life coach who specializes in helping women build the life they deserve by asking for what they want without shame and loving who they are without reserve.

She plans on starting a revolution. You can read more about her at www.DarlingPropaganda.com.

www.ingramcontent.com/pod-product-compliance
Lightning Source LLC
Chambersburg PA
CBHW022102280326
41933CB00007B/226